FIRESIDE

Also by Rachel Carr:

Stepping Stones to Japanese Floral Art
A Year of Flowers
Hours and Flowers
Japanese Floral Art: Symbolism, Cult & Practice
The Japanese Way with Flowers
The Picture Story of Japan
Creative Ways with Flowers: The Best of Two Worlds, East and West
Yoga . . . Today! (record album)

YOGA

FOR ALL AGES

Rachel E. Carr

A Fireside Book Published by Simon and Schuster

My gratitude to all the children and teen-agers who posed for the yoga exercises in this book. They appear on the following pages:

Gail Bendheim—90 bottom left, 91 top, 92, 95 top
Leslie Best—117, 126, 127 top left
André Bossier—116 rear
Julie Davis—86 center, 89
Nancy Edwards—87 top, 88 top left and bottom, 93
Gerrit Folsom—86 bottom, 90 bottom right, 95 bottom, 96
Nancy Frankel—87 center and bottom, 90 top, 91 bottom
Bill Hilson—88 top right
Dwight Hilson—86 top, 94
Melissa Hilson—123, 138-39 top
Kim Hober—118 top left, 124, 125
Joyce Kennedy—118 top right, 120
Kim Larkin—133 right, 136 bottom
Jill Levine—135, 136 top, 138-39 bottom
Mark Levine—118 bottom right, 122, 134
Robert Linde—121 right
Philip MacGregor—127 top right, 133 left and center, 137
Yukari Morimoto—118 bottom left, 127 bottom, 130-31
Tod Phillips—121 left, 132
Elizabeth Rees—119, 128
Tom Rees—116 front, 129, 140

SBN 671-21019-X Casebound
SBN 671-22151-5 Paperback
Library of Congress Catalog Card Number: 78-189739
Designed by Libra Graphics, Inc.
Manufactured in the United States of America

1 2 3 4 5 6 7 8 9 10

For Ed

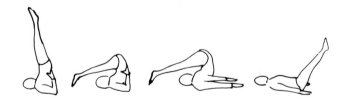

Contents

Acknowledgments

Seldom is a book published without the help of others, and it is here that I wish to express my gratitude to those who helped create *Yoga for All Ages.*

Family Circle magazine has provided many of the pictures taken of me by George Nordhausen; John R. Kennedy patiently photographed a major portion of this book, and has been particularly successful in capturing the children in different yoga postures. And I am especially grateful to Katy Hilson, a longtime student of mine and a serious follower of yoga, for generously contributing her talent in photography.

My early discussions with Camille Davied and Fay Kramer were most helpful in the preparation of this book.

My husband, Ed, was of invaluable assistance in supplying comments on the text from the masculine viewpoint, and also in testing and timing each exercise.

PHOTO CREDITS

KATY HILSON: photos on pages 25, 32, 40, 56, 57, 67, 70 *top,* 76, 86 *top,* 87, 88, 90 *top* and *bottom left,* 91, 92-94, 95 *top,* 116, 119, 128, 129, 138 *top,* 139 *top,* 140, 145.

JOHN R. KENNEDY: photos on pages 24, 33, 37, 41-45, 48, 49, 54, 55, 58-63, 69, 77-83, 86 *bottom,* 89, 90 *bottom right,* 95 *bottom,* 96, 117, 118, 120, 122-127, 130, 131, 133-137, 138 *bottom,* 139 *bottom,* 142.

EDWARD N. KIMBALL, JR.: photos on pages 121 and 132.

GEORGE NORDHAUSEN OF *Family Circle:* photos on pages 22, 23, 26-28, 34-36, 46, 47, 50, 51, 66, 70 *bottom,* 71-73, 98-112.

Introduction

We are all seeking some magic formula for good health and inner peace in a world that is charged with tension and anxiety. How do we find it? The answer is not simple, but there is a way. Through yoga.

In the past ten years, yoga has been making astonishing inroads in the American way of life. Why this surge of interest in an Indian science of physical and mental health that is over five thousand years old? Obviously its fundamental principles have something to offer, for in every large city one can always find yoga instruction—at yoga centers, at the YMCA and YWCA, at country clubs, and even in department stores.

What is yoga all about? Let me begin by defining it in simple terms and separating its practical aspects from the metaphysical.

Essentially, yoga is a search for health and well-being on two levels: physical and spiritual. It is an art of living that holds the key to youthfulness, vitality, and long life. It leads to harmony and peace of mind. Its age-old teachings apply with special urgency to our needs for a calmer, healthier way of life today when tension is the number one killer in our society. It is needed especially by productive people who have achieved some measure of success but who continue to go through life plagued by tension. It works for people of all ages and all walks of life. I have been helped immeasurably by yoga, in ways that I shall describe. I have also observed its effects on others, and have seen it produce results that could have been achieved in no other way.

A successful friend of mine who had won many tributes in the business world is a typical example. She lived on tranquilizers. "This is how I let down," she said. "In my world I simply can't find the time to exercise or even relax."

"Have you ever thought of taking up yoga?" I asked.

"Heavens, no! Eastern mysticism isn't for me. Besides, I'm too stiff to sit in the Lotus pose or stand on my head."

"There is much more to yoga," I told her, "than the mystical side or even the more difficult physical exercises. You could learn simple breathing that brings oxygen to your lungs to open up a reservoir of energy. You could do limbering and stretching exercises to release tension, and quiet contemplation would bring you mental poise. Can't you spare twenty to thirty minutes a day for that?"

She hesitated. "I suppose it's worth a try."

It was indeed worth a try. As the weeks passed, my jumpy, irritable friend, under the practice of yoga, transformed herself into a more poised and relaxed woman. Sans tranquilizers, pep pills, or sleeping tablets. It was from my varied experiences with other women—and with men and teen-agers and children, too—that the idea for this book grew.

I wish to emphasize that yoga has no theology. Although it often leads to a religious outlook, its doctrines do not supplant our own religious beliefs but rather intensify them. For those who lack the comfort of religion, yoga brings urgently needed inner peace by showing man how to develop his capacities to their utmost.

I am speaking now not of yoga in the mysterious Eastern sense, which often confuses the Western mind, but of yoga expressly adapted to Western living. It is not an experimental science; the facts are on record. It is a comprehensive philosophy with different paths or divisions. Those best suited to Western living are Hatha yoga—devoted to physical well-being—and its counterpart Raja, or mental, yoga. It is therefore more than a means to achieve physical fitness.

Yoga is truly for all ages. It has something unique to contribute at every age level. During the tender years of a child's life—beginning at about age five—yoga can help build muscle strength and establish good breathing habits and good posture. Children find yoga great fun, and parents will enjoy introducing them to the exercises for children in Chapter 5. Besides being suited to the wonderful flexibility that most children possess, those exercises that resemble animals, birds and insects are, I find, appealing to a child's imagination and evoke a natural and enthusiastic response in young yoga practitioners.

Chapter 2—A Yoga Course in Six Stages—is really the heart of the book. It offers exercises that are suitable for the limber and not so limber. Each stage is based on a gradual buildup in stretching, toning, deep breathing and relaxing. No hard-and-fast time schedule is given for the stages, because the number of days required for each depends on individual physical fitness. Some people are ready to move on to the next stage after a week; others take a little longer.

Teen-agers have followed this course with positive results. Girls who struggle with a weight problem or lack physical grace have found the exercises a way to self-improvement; boys have used the yoga breathing techniques in track and swimming, and the muscle-control exercises have given them additional physical stamina. The teen-agers who posed for the exercises in Chapter 3 have had no more than a few weeks of yoga.

It is of interest that a number of medical books on natural childbirth advocate yoga breathing and physical exercises during pregnancy. One of my students, who had kept physically fit through yoga during her pregnancy, proudly announced that by breathing the yoga way and knowing how to relax, she was able to experience the final stage of delivery of her first baby with a sense of joy. She was forty.

Men often hesitate to admit that they practice yoga. "It's not quite the thing other men expect of me" is the general feeling. Yet faithful followers realize that yoga helps to prolong youth, relax tension, and bring the good looks that come with well-being.

Yoga has also reached into the lives of the elderly, who respond quickly to its spiritual as well as its physical aspects. One of my students at eighty-six enjoys all the breathing exercises synchronized with the stretching and limbering movements. "I feel like a running stream," she remarked cheerfully one day. "It's mainly the meditation that has brought my spirit alive again."

She became so enthusiastic about the benefits of yoga that she has organized a group of her friends who meet twice a week. "We have our own yoga sessions," she said. "The exercises we enjoy most are the ones we can do sitting in a chair. I'm so glad you've included them in your book."

A student of mine in her late seventies was crippled with arthritis. Little could be done for her, and her increasing incapacity resulted in severe depression. She sought the help of psychiatry and was told that she was behaving like a squirrel trapped in a cage, going round and round without escape. "Learn to grow old gracefully and accept your disabilities," she was advised. This sent her into a deeper depression. She indeed felt trapped.

We began with deep-breathing exercises and quiet stretching and limbering movements, which she was able to enjoy for the first time. With the help of concentration exercises, she gradually learned how to unload the burden of fear that weighed her down. She looked forward to small pleasures that did not exhaust her physically. She made a careful accounting of her daily activities, which were punctuated with such positive actions as writing a letter to a friend, reading a good book, attending a ballet, and doing things for others. Then came the short periods of mental calm she experienced through daily meditation.

Learning to relax and let go is a vital part of yoga practice. Chapter 6 is devoted entirely to Simple Steps to Relaxing. The mind-sharpening exercises and ways to attain mind control are explained in Chapter 7, Yoga for the Mind.

Many yoga enthusiasts in the Western world who practice Hatha yoga — the physical postures and breathing — have avoided Raja yoga — the spiritual counterpart — mainly because the language often used to describe the meditation and the exercises for mental discipline seems mystical. As a result, the underlying concepts are rejected as being "too Eastern" and not applicable to the West. On the contrary, yoga meditation is a simple, straightforward mental exercise which adds immeasurably to one's sense of inner peace and makes the practice of physical yoga much more pleasurable.

After all, the concept of meditation is not exclusively an Eastern one. It is an integral part of Western religions; and meditation, in one form or another, is within the experience of most of us. Perhaps we have gained a feeling of peace by sitting quietly on a hilltop or by the seashore simply reflecting on the world around us.

Actually, at such times we are engaging in meditation.

In yoga, meditation has been taken out of the realm of the occasional and chance occurrence. It is acknowledged as an important aspect of human existence, and yoga has developed ways to achieve a rewarding state of meditation. It is these formal methods that Westerners find difficult to practice and are reluctant to accept. Furthermore, the expressions used carry to the Western mind connotations of the supernatural and the mystical. Consequently, many people are put off, not realizing that there are no adequate words to convey the meaning. Once one gets beyond the language and into meditation itself, there is no need for words. The experience will provide the explanation.

For many of us, yoga has proved to be a magic formula for good health and inner peace — a magic within the reach of anyone who is willing to make yoga a part of vital living.

Rachel E. Carr

Chapter

1

YOGA, A WAY OF LIFE

When India's late Prime Minister Nehru was asked how he managed to keep calm as tempers flared in political arenas, he replied, "It's simple. When the going is rough, I meditate."

Yoga's guidelines have helped and influenced not only such great men of the East as Nehru and Gandhi, but also many well-known personalities of the West.

The noted violinist Yehudi Menuhin says that in order of values he places sleep and yoga exercises before the practice of the violin. Ski champion Jean-Claude Killy was photographed practicing yoga before the world championships at Portillo, Chile, where he won two gold medals. Free diver Jacques Mayol spent hours in the Lotus pose at the bottom of a 17-foot tank practicing deep yoga breathing until he could hold his breath for four minutes and two seconds. He achieved a world-record depth in free diving.

Other serious followers of yoga with widely diversified backgrounds are ageless movie stars Gloria Swanson, Greta Garbo, and Cary Grant; dress designer Pauline Trigère; dancer Ruth St. Denis; former middleweight champion Sugar Ray Robinson; opera singer Robert Merrill; artist Peter Max; golfer Gary Player; and Israel's David Ben-Gurion.

There is a yoga camp in the Laurentian mountains of Val Morin, Quebec, which attracts hundreds of people every year from different parts of the world. But one does not have far to travel for yoga instruction. Most large cities in the United States have qualified instructors, many of whom come from India. In New York City the well-known yogi Vithaldas, with whom I have studied for some years, has taught a range of people that includes overworked executives, secretaries, models, and famous personalities, among them Yehudi Menuhin, Gladys Swarthout, and Arlene Francis.

Yogi Vithaldas says his greatest rewards in teaching yoga have come from the students whom he influenced and who changed their lives by giving up smoking, heavy drinking, and the use of drugs. The secret of keeping physically and mentally fit, he believes, is to practice yoga exercises and a little meditation every day, even if it is only for 10 to 15 minutes.

Commenting on the extraordinary ability of yoga to control bodily func-

tions, a medical article* reported on experiments at Harvard Medical School in which every one of the twenty volunteers was able to achieve small but nevertheless significant changes in his blood pressure. This remarkable series of experiments offers hope that man may someday regulate his blood pressure, heart rate, and internal organs by direct command of his conscious brain.

In a more recent experiment† involving dedicated Zen and yogi meditators, it was evidenced that the meditators were indeed capable of asserting mind over matter. Researchers wired them to electroencephalograph (EEG) machines and found that the meditators could by sheer force of will, due to years of training, produce "profound trance states, raise and lower blood pressure, reduce body temperature, slow heart rates and, in general, tap into physiological functions thought to be forever beyond the reach of conscious control."

Even though interest in the science of yoga is widespread, perhaps none is more misunderstood. Its teachings are sometimes confused with yogurt, yogi, judo and karate—of which the last two are arts of self-defense.

A yogi (feminine, yogini) is simply one who practices yoga. Yoga, in essence, symbolizes the unity of body, mind and spirit. Anyone can practice it and choose the path of its disciplines that best suits his own needs. Many of today's followers limit their practice to the acquiring of physical health. Others seek the comfort, sense of secu-

* Fred Warshofsky, "Visceral Control: Science Goes Yoga." *Family Health,* April 1970.
† David M. Rovik, "Brain Waves." *Look* magazine, October 6, 1970.

14

rity, and peace of mind that come from meditation. A few go on to the deeper spiritual pursuits.

EARLY BEGINNINGS OF YOGA

The tradition of yoga began in northern India over five thousand years ago among a learned aristocratic society of philosophers, scholars, and warriors who examined the ephemeral quality of life, with its inevitable sufferings and tragedies, and sought to give it deeper meaning and purpose. These principles grew into a tradition of practice and culture, and were first formulated into a science of physical and mental health by the Indian philosopher Patanjali, in about the second century B.C.

When yoga was adopted by the Brahmins, a priestly caste, its doctrines were incorporated into the Hindu faith and were made part of its scriptures as a method of attaining union with God. The word *yoga* comes from the Sanskrit root *yuj*, meaning "union" or "yoke" — to connote a union of the individual soul with the Divine Spirit.

There are different yoga paths or training methods, all of which lead to the highest spiritual development. This book is concerned only with the fundamentals of the two that are best suited to Western living: Hatha yoga (the way of physical training to prepare the mind and body for meditation), and Raja yoga (the way of meditation). In a strict sense, Raja yoga includes Hatha yoga.

The other paths, less known to the Western world, are Karma yoga (the way of right action); Bhakti yoga (the way of devotion); Jnana yoga (the way of knowledge through man's intellectual pursuit); Mantra yoga (the way of inner communion through chanting words of power); and Kundalini yoga (the way of arousing latent powers to produce illumination through breathing and concentration on the vital nerve plexuses in the spine and head).

The highest stage in yoga, to which very few aspire, is *Samadhi*, or enlightenment. Patanjali, in his *Yoga Sutras* (teachings), describes the different stages to be followed on the path to enlightenment. They include ten rules of the yoga code of morality, with restraints and observances, similar to the Judeo-Christian Ten Commandments (*Yama-Niyama*); physical postures (*Asanas*); breath control (*Pranayama*); nerve control (*Pratyahara*); concentration (*Dharana*); meditation (*Dhyana*); enlightenment (*Samadhi*).

Though our life-style in the West is not conducive to a dedicated spiritual search for enlightenment as it is practiced in the East, we may, through the study of yoga, become nourished inwardly by keeping spiritually tuned up. Since yoga is a philosophy of living, with its help we can become more effectively active than we had been without it. We can expect a high degree of responsiveness from a healthy body brought under the discipline of the mind. Our energies are directed to the creative and the constructive and away from distractions. Consequently, we can achieve a greater sense of freedom and serenity.

Chapter

2

A YOGA COURSE IN SIX STAGES

Everyone talks about exercise, but relatively few of us do anything about it. Yet we know our muscles must be used to maintain a healthy life.

Since nature made our bodies for constant action in walking, bending and climbing, our muscles become rigid when we do not use them. The great advantage of yoga exercises is that they bring all the muscle groups into play. This means the range of movement can be increased in the muscles, tendons and ligaments and the joints they support, with particular emphasis on stretching the spine to increase its flexibility. Physical poise is developed through the yoga postures, which in themselves are a series of supple, graceful movements. Some of the postures may appear deceptively relaxed, but in reality they are dynamic. The muscles are slowly stretched to full length and then the postures are held in perfect stillness, causing blood to flow evenly throughout the body.

With the improvement of muscle

tone and flexibility of the joints and spine, sluggish and aging glands are revitalized. Furthermore, the yoga poses (in particular the Plow, Bow, Cobra, Locust, Shoulderstand, Headstand and Fish, which are given in this book) not only strengthen weak back muscles and improve the posture, but also act directly on the endocrine glands that influence sexual function. When our body is relaxed, supple and well toned, we become free to enjoy more complete sexual expression.

Through yoga we also learn that deep controlled breathing is nature's tranquilizer and rejuvenator. Singers, actors and athletes know the value, indeed the necessity, of controlled breathing. It has many beneficial effects. By slowing down the rate of respiration, it reduces strain on the heart. Its stimulating action improves the metabolism, transforming deposits of fat into body fuel. By keeping the lungs well exercised, it increases their resistance to the common cold and other respiratory ailments. By providing sufficient oxygen to the body, it wards off fatigue and sluggishness.

When we breathe deeply, we increase the supply of oxygen into the bloodstream and hence into the muscles, joints and organs of the body. This process increases the ability of the muscles to respond and raises the level of energy.

Most of the breathing exercises in yoga are done through the nose with the mouth closed. The reason: our nose acts as a vacuum cleaner, which sweeps in with the air fine particles of dust and bacteria. When air enters the nostrils, it passes through a labyrinth of filters that screens out dust and bacteria and warms the air before it reaches our lungs. When we exhale through the nostrils, rather than through the mouth, our lungs gain stamina, since they take a longer time to deflate.

Few of us are consciously aware of how our emotions influence the way we breathe. When we are excited, our heart beats faster and breathing takes on a staccato-like rhythm. When we are depressed, our body slumps and breathing becomes an effort. But when we are happy we stand to full height, the face is calm, and breathing is deeper and easier. If we breathe as nature intended, by expanding our lungs to full capacity, we can revitalize our energy, calm our nerves, induce restful sleep—and live longer.

The practice of yoga alone will not increase or decrease weight. Only diet can do that. But through yoga you will lose inches as your muscles are toned and body weight is redistributed. If you have a weight problem, either over or under your normal poundage, take a look at what you eat. Are your meals nutritionally sound? Follow a balanced diet either to lose or to gain. Drink plenty of water—about eight glasses a day: this is the number-one purifying agent for the body. *The best prescription for good health is daily exercise, enough rest, and the right diet.*

Realize that it is never too late to start looking and feeling younger. You can slow down the aging process by caring for yourself, especially during the dangerous middle years when you are inclined to eat more and exercise less.

When you begin this yoga course, establish a daily routine. Set aside 30 minutes a day, either at one time or divided if it is more convenient. *Yoga should be done slowly, with frequent rests to replenish inner reserve.*

The best time to practice is early in the morning, before you are caught up in the day's activities. If before breakfast is impracticable, choose any convenient time when you can have quiet and privacy—before lunch or dinner, in midafternoon or before bedtime. Find a well-ventilated area. Silence the phone and close the door so that you can tune in to the harmony of your body and mind. If you prefer to exercise out of doors, select a shady, temperate place away from wind or excessive heat.

Before doing any exercises, wait at least two hours after a heavy meal, an hour after a light snack. Exercising too soon after a meal may cause nausea.

Wear a swimsuit or a leotard to give you freedom of movement; for men, undershorts or swim trunks.

It is best to exercise on a firm but not hard surface. A towel spread over a heavy rug, or three to four folded blankets, will give you a comfortable support. If you wish to make your own yoga mat, use compressed foam rubber, or padded cotton 2″ thick, measuring 36″ × 72″, and cover it with a washable slip-on case. This is similar to the traditional Indian yoga mat.

After the first few days of practice you may experience some stiffness in the muscles, but this will disappear with gradual toning and limbering. You might enjoy starting this course with a group of friends. Meeting once or twice a week and sharing your yoga experiences will spur you on to regular daily practice on your own.

To use this book, read the instructions for each exercise before beginning, so that you can follow it easily. Keep the book within reach, open to the picture, to refer to when in doubt.

HOW TO GET THE MOST OUT OF
THIS BASIC YOGA COURSE

If you are limber enough, you will find that the exercises given in each stage can be done within a week, but *please don't rush through the stages*. Even though some of the exercises may appear too simple for you, they are included for a reason. To gain maximum benefit from each exercise, it should be done slowly and smoothly.

If you are not so limber or haven't been exercising, do each stage for an extra three days or more before moving on to the next stage. Skip the exercises that are beyond your physical capacity, or attempt them as best you can. Don't try to perfect each exercise before moving on to the next; you will only become frustrated. It will take time before your body becomes limber enough to do the exercises with ease and control. With continued practice, you will be surprised to find that those exercises which once seemed impossible to do will become less difficult. Remember that to gain the benefits of yoga you don't have to do the more complicated exercises, such as assuming the Lotus pose, that demand greater flexibility of the legs, or to

acquire ultimate balance, as in the Head-stand. Take the course slowly, to give your muscles time to stretch and tone; otherwise you will end up with muscle strain.

The exercises for each stage have been timed to help you pace your practice period. Since each stage does not extend beyond 10 minutes a day, take an extra 10 minutes to review previous lessons and practice those exercises which are still a challenge. Spend at least 5 minutes a day, or the additional time of your 30 minutes, in a little quiet contemplation and relaxation. You will find many helpful suggestions in Chapter 6, Simple Steps to Relaxing, and Chapter 7, Yoga for the Mind.

As a safety measure, before you begin this course consult your doctor if you are suffering from any internal disorder, high or low blood pressure, or a weak heart. In all probability, the exercises given for limbering, stretching and deep breathing will improve your health.

You are now ready to embark on your first step to yoga.

Summary of the First Stage

Exercise Time: 10 Minutes

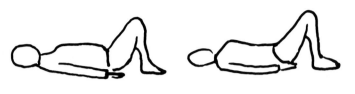

ABDOMINAL BREATHING

Stretches lower lobes of lungs; calms emotions; induces restful sleep.

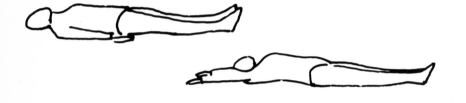

COMPLETE BREATHING

Exercises lungs fully; tones up entire circulatory system; gives body renewed energy.

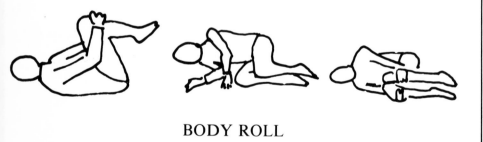

BODY ROLL

Releases body tension; tones hips and thighs.

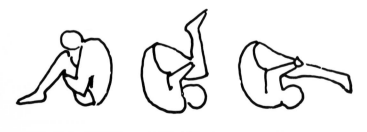

ROCKING THE SPINE

Limbers stiff spine; excellent warm-up for entire body.

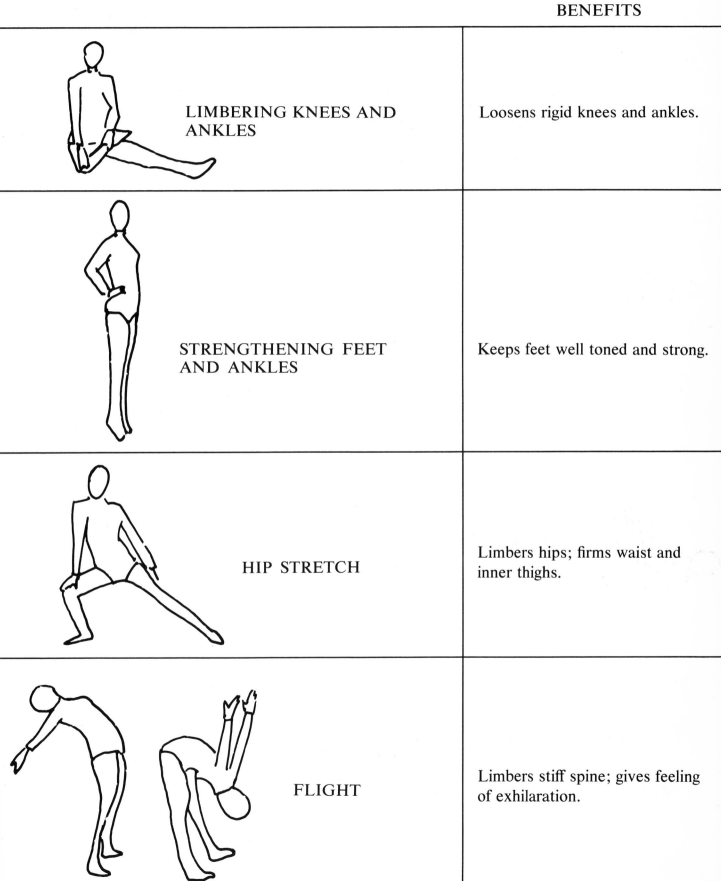

LIMBERING KNEES AND ANKLES	Loosens rigid knees and ankles.
STRENGTHENING FEET AND ANKLES	Keeps feet well toned and strong.
HIP STRETCH	Limbers hips; firms waist and inner thighs.
FLIGHT	Limbers stiff spine; gives feeling of exhilaration.

FIRST STEPS TO YOGA BREATHING

1. ABDOMINAL BREATHING

The key to diaphragmatic breathing is simple: *as you inhale, expand the abdomen (blow it out like a balloon); as you exhale, contract the abdomen (pull it in toward the spine).*

Think of the inflow and outflow of your breath as a silken thread, so that you have the feeling of a smooth flow.

The purpose of Abdominal Breathing is to stretch the lower lobes of the lungs. The chest is kept still. This type of quiet breathing will calm emotions and induce restful sleep.

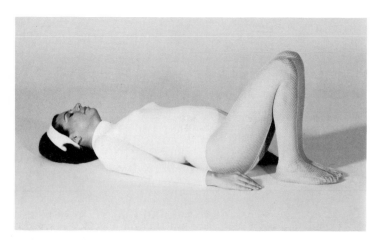

Lie on your back with legs bent, feet close to buttocks, eyes closed. Inhale, expanding the abdomen while keeping the chest still.

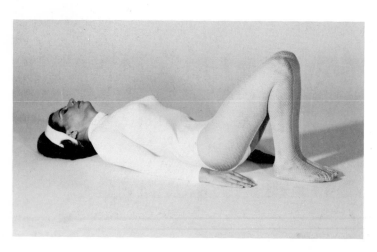

Exhale, pulling in the abdomen and drawing it back to the spine. Repeat 5 times, following this ratio:

Inhale: 5 seconds (expand
       abdomen)
Exhale: 10 seconds (contract
       abdomen)

2. COMPLETE BREATHING

In Complete Breathing, air is pulled up from the abdomen into the rib cage and chest to fully inflate the lungs. The flow of breath should be deep, smooth and rhythmic, yet its vigorous action will stimulate circulation and give the body renewed strength.

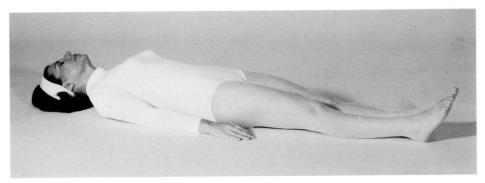

Lie on your back with legs together, arms by your sides, palms down. Close your eyes. Inhale, expanding the abdomen a little, then pull air up into the rib cage and chest. Your abdomen will automatically be drawn in as the ribs move out and chest expands.

Exhale, slowly letting your breath out in a smooth, continuous flow until the abdomen is drawn in and the rib cage and chest are relaxed. Repeat three times. The process of inhalation and exhalation should take about 10 seconds.

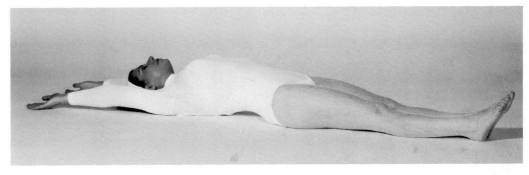

Next, breathe in as in Step 1 but raise your arms overhead till back of hands touches the floor. Hold your breath for 10–15 seconds (the longer the better) and stretch like a cat from head to toe. Then slowly release the air as you drop your arms forward and down to the sides. Repeat three times.

3. BODY ROLL

Rolling from side to side is a good way to firm thighs and hips, and to release tension knots in the back and shoulders.

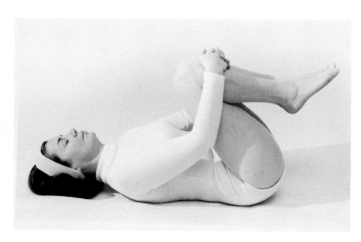

Lie on your back; clasp hands around bent knees and press them firmly toward chest. Close your eyes. Inhale deeply, at the same time rolling over to your right.

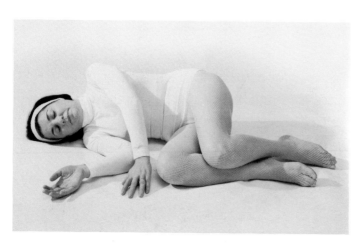

As you drop limply to the floor, exhale completely; release arms and legs. Relax for 5 seconds to feel tension knots dissolving.

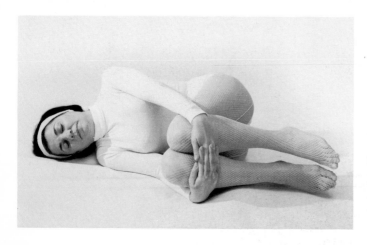

While on your right side, clasp hands around bent knees. Inhale deeply. With right elbow push yourself up and over to your left side, exhaling as you drop limply to the floor. Let go again and relax for 5 seconds. Repeat cycle three times, rolling from left to right, then right to left.

4. ROCKING THE SPINE

The rapid movements of rocking back and forth are a warm-up to stretch the spine and stimulate circulation. You should experience a surge of energy throughout your body. But if your spine is rigid, you may find the rapid movements startling and a little difficult. Don't rush into this exercise. Take it gradually. It may be weeks before you will be able to get your legs over your head with toes touching the floor.

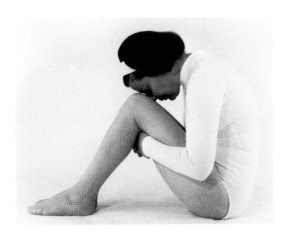

Sit with hands clasped under bent knees, head down. Keep back well rounded, knees to forehead. *Fingers remain interlocked throughout the exercise.*

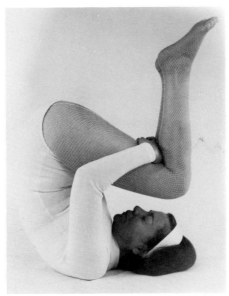

Inhale, rock back a little, then exhale and rock forward with head close to knees.

Continue to rock back and forth; each time stretch legs a little farther over head until toes touch the floor, or as far as they will reach. Repeat rocking motion 10 times. Then relax completely, breathing quietly and deeply.

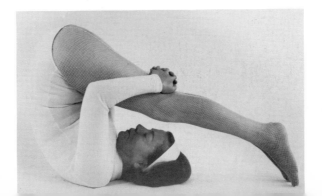

5. LIMBERING KNEES AND ANKLES

This preliminary stretching exercise will restore elasticity to stiff knees and ankles, and will prepare you for the sitting yoga postures, such as the Perfect, Half-Lotus and Lotus. At first your knees may stubbornly rest in the air, but with practice they will limber.

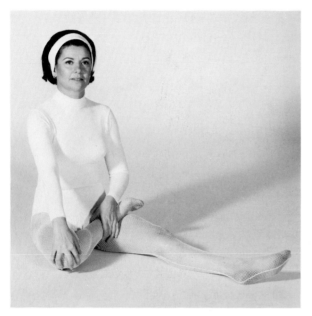

Sit with legs apart, spine straight, arms to your sides. Bend right leg so that foot rests on left thigh, heel close to crotch. Grasp right knee with right hand and right ankle with left hand. Gently press knee down to the floor, or as far as possible without straining. Hold for 5 seconds, release knee, then press down again. Repeat 5 times. Bounce leg lightly to increase circulation.

Repeat same movements with left leg. The longer you are able to hold knee down, the better.

For an additional exercise in limbering legs see Exercise 78 (step 2).

STRENGTHENING FEET AND ANKLES

This exercise can be done anywhere with shoes off. It strengthens arches and ankles, and relieves aching, tired and swollen feet.

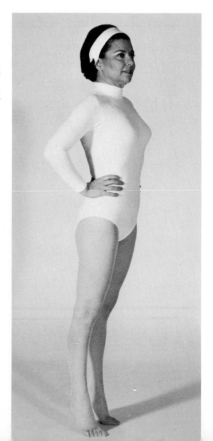

Stand on a firm surface with feet together, hands on hips. Inhale, rise up on toes, balance for 5 seconds to feel pull in the arches and ankles. Exhale, lower heels. Repeat 5 times.
Then rise on toes. Slowly rotate feet to outer sides, back on heels to inner sides, and return to tiptoe position. Repeat 5 times.

For additional exercises in strengthening feet and ankles see Exercise 74.

6. HIP STRETCH

Hard-to-tone inner thighs will get their workout in the Hip Stretch. It is also a limbering and toning exercise for the waist and legs.

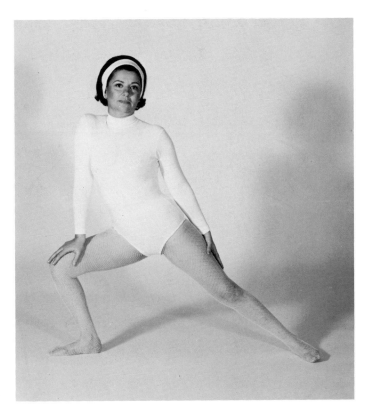

Stand with feet far apart, hands on thighs, spine straight. Turn right foot out; bend the knee with right hand resting on it. Stretch left leg away from you till knee is perfectly straight with left hand on side of thigh. Inhale and hold for 5 seconds; at the same time press right hand on right knee and contract inner thigh muscles. Exhale; return to standing position, keeping legs apart. Repeat three times. Repeat same movements bending left knee.

7. FLIGHT

To get the feeling of flight, imagine that you are about to soar up into the clouds as your arms are thrust backward and forward in rhythmic motion. These limbering movements, synchronized with breathing, will loosen stiff back and shoulder muscles, at the same time exercising the lungs.

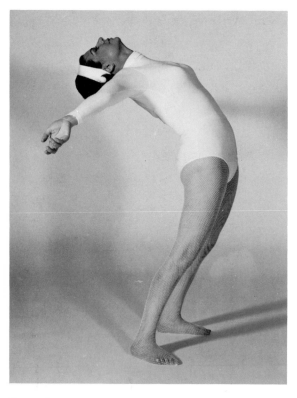

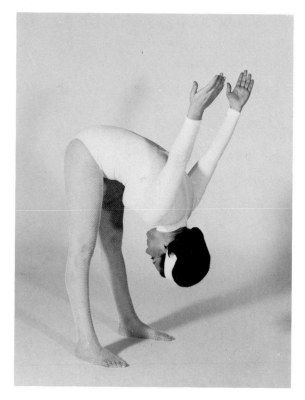

Stand with feet apart, arms outstretched at sides. Close your eyes. Inhale and bend as far back as possible with arms thrust back. Hold for 5 seconds.

Exhale; bend forward and down, keeping arms back and up, with neck limp. Hold for 5 seconds. Inhale and bend backward again. Repeat the same movements three times, increasing the backward and forward stretches.

This concludes the first stage in yoga. You should already be feeling more relaxed and limber. Before you conclude your daily practice, take a few extra minutes to lie on your back with eyes closed and entertain only pleasant thoughts that will establish a happier mood for the rest of the day.

Much is written about the power of the breath in the ancient Indian scriptures of the *Upanishads*. There is a delightful parable which describes a dispute among the powers of the body, each claiming its indispensable force. The powers finally agreed that to prove their worth, each would take leave of the body individually to judge how the other powers would survive.

The eyes were the first to depart. On returning after a year's absence, they asked, "How have you lived without us?"

And the powers replied, "Like blind people we have lived. Not seeing with the eyes, but breathing with the breath, speaking with the tongue, hearing with the ears, knowing with the mind, and generating with the seed. Thus have we lived."

When the ears departed and returned, the powers gave this answer: "Like deaf people we have lived, but with the help of all the others we have been able to exist."

Then the tongue took leave, and it was given a similar answer on its return: "Like dumb people we have lived, but we have managed by pulling forces together."

Next the mind took leave of the body. For a year the powers struggled. "We have lived like fools without you," they told the mind, "but we were able to exist, for we all stood united."

The departure of the seed caused the body and mind great anguish. "Without you we have been barren, for in no way were we able to bear fruit of the womb," they said, "but we have managed to exist."

Now it was time for the breath to take leave of the body. But the breath warned the other powers, saying, "Gentlemen, don't deceive yourselves. It is I alone dividing myself fivefold who keep together this body and support it."

But the powers insisted that the breath be tested. Just as the breath rose and appeared to be leaving, the body was torn apart.

"Sir," the powers cried, "don't leave us! You are indeed the supreme ruler of us all."

The yogis call the energy we absorb through deep breathing *prana*, meaning "life force."

Summary of the Second Stage

Exercise Time: 10 Minutes

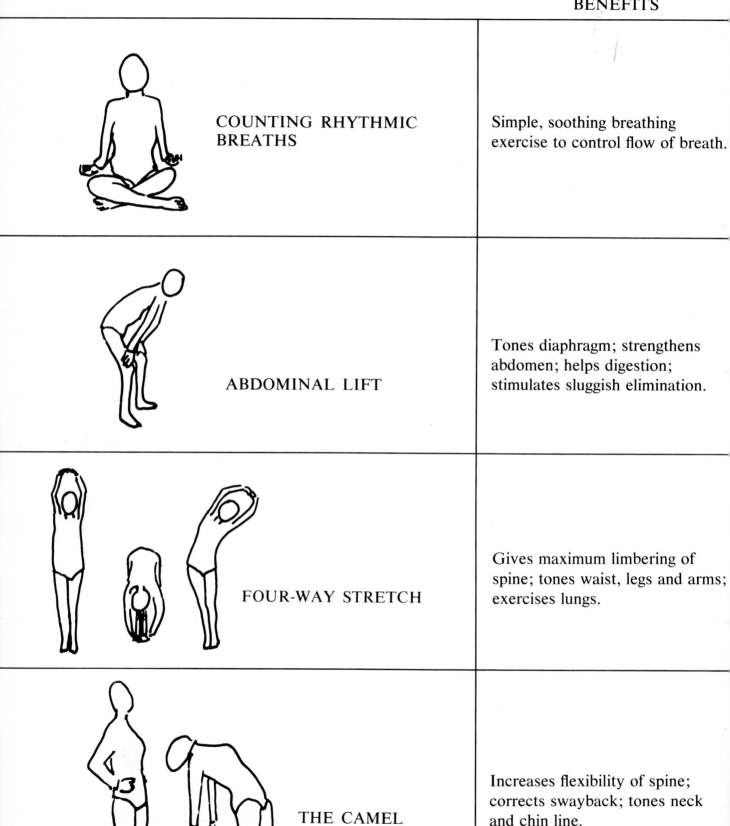

COUNTING RHYTHMIC BREATHS	Simple, soothing breathing exercise to control flow of breath.
ABDOMINAL LIFT	Tones diaphragm; strengthens abdomen; helps digestion; stimulates sluggish elimination.
FOUR-WAY STRETCH	Gives maximum limbering of spine; tones waist, legs and arms; exercises lungs.
THE CAMEL	Increases flexibility of spine; corrects swayback; tones neck and chin line.

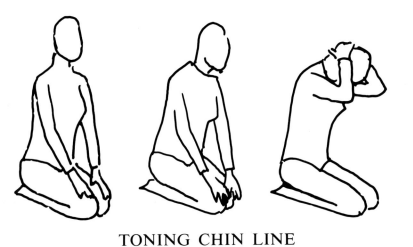

TONING CHIN LINE AND LIMBERING NECK

Decreases double chin and folds in neck. Loosens tight muscles in back of neck and shoulders.

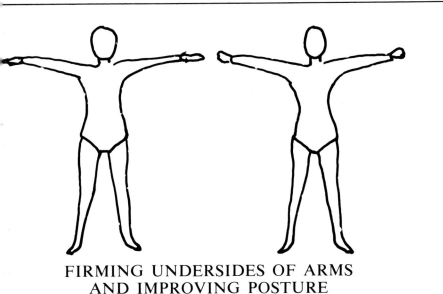

FIRMING UNDERSIDES OF ARMS AND IMPROVING POSTURE

Firms flabby undersides of arms; improves posture; exercises lungs.

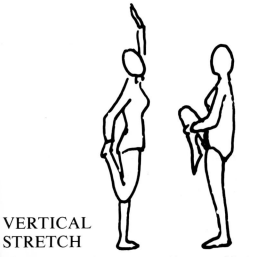

BALANCING EXERCISES

Improves posture, balance, and power of concentration.

VERTICAL STRETCH

KNEE BEND

8. COUNTING RHYTHMIC BREATHS

Good posture is important during breathing. Your spine should be kept straight but not rigid. If you hunch as you breathe, this will hinder the expansion of your lungs. To avoid distraction, close your eyes and concentrate on the point between the eyebrows. Think only of the rhythmic flow of your breath, and gently dismiss any straying thoughts that invade your mind. This is easier said than done, but it does come with practice.

Most breathing exercises in yoga are done in a meditative sitting posture, such as the Easy Posture shown for this exercise. Legs are loosely crossed, spine is straight, and hands rest on the knees with palms up, fingers relaxed. If this is not a comfortable position for you, sit in a chair with your legs slightly apart and feet flat on the floor. Keep your spine straight and your eyes closed.

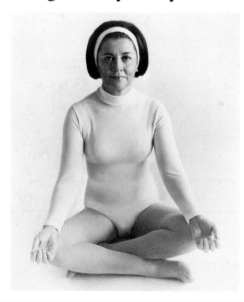

To the count of 5 seconds inhale deeply and smoothly, fully inflating the lungs.

Hold your breath for 10 seconds with the mind concentrating on the force of energy you are drawing into your body.

To the count of 10 seconds, exhale smoothly.

Repeat three times without stopping. Gradually increase the retention time until you are able to hold breath in for 20 seconds.

9. ABDOMINAL LIFT

The great advantage of the Abdominal Lift is that it can be done in different positions: *standing* as shown at right with body bent slightly forward and legs apart; *sitting in a chair* with legs apart and heels flat on the floor (Exercise 65); *lying flat* with legs bent and apart or sitting cross-legged on the floor (Exercise 44).

Try this exercise first in the standing position, hands above knees.

10. FOUR-WAY STRETCH

To gain maximum benefit from the Four-way stretch, hold each movement for 2 seconds.

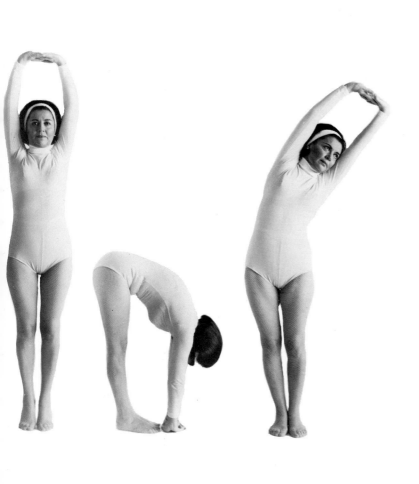

First, stand with feet together, hands to the sides. Inhale deeply and raise arms overhead. Interlock fingers, palms up. Hold breath and stretch upward on tiptoe, feeling pull in the spine and undersides of arms.

Second, exhale and bend forward, touching the floor if possible, with clasped hands. Bring them close to feet, or as far down as you can.

Third, inhale and come up to standing position with arms raised. Hold breath. Bend to the left and to the right without bending elbows. Hold each time to feel pull along the sides, then stretch upward on tiptoe. Lower arms. Exhale and relax.

Repeat twice.

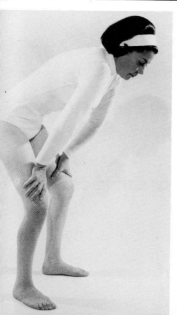

Inhale deeply through the nose; then vigorously exhale through the mouth in a "ha" sound. This will empty the lungs and create a vacuum in the abdominal cavity. Hold your breath and draw up the diaphragm, pressing it against the rib cage, so that the abdomen is pulled in and up toward the back of the spine. Hold from 5 to 10 seconds without breathing. Relax. Repeat three times.

When the abdominal muscles have been strengthened through the lift (this may take two to three weeks), practice the pumping movement by pulling in the abdominal muscles, then forcefully thrusting them out 5 to 10 times while holding the breath. Repeat three times.

33

11. THE CAMEL

If your spine is stiff, take this exercise in two stages to gradually limber the muscles. Bend only as far back as you can without straining. With continued practice you will increase the elasticity of your spine.

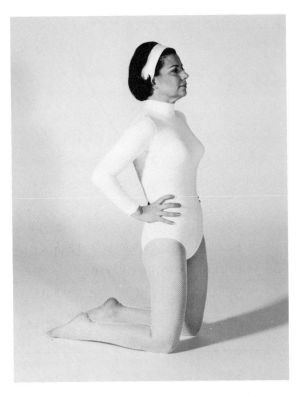

Kneel with legs apart, hands on hips. Close your eyes. Inhale while bending slightly backward. Hold for 5 seconds. (If you are unable to hold your breath in this position, breathe freely.) Exhale as you return to the upright position.

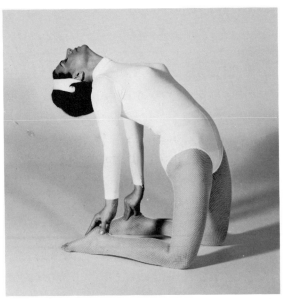

Inhale while bending backward reaching for your heels or ankles. Breathe freely and hold this pose from 5 to 10 seconds. Exhale and slowly return to the kneeling position. Repeat three times.

Variations of The Camel are shown in Exercises 45 and 85.

12. TONING CHIN LINE AND LIMBERING NECK

These exercises can also be done in a chair if the kneeling position is uncomfortable. Sit with legs together and feet flat on floor, spine straight. Kneeling, however, will increase the flexibility of the legs.

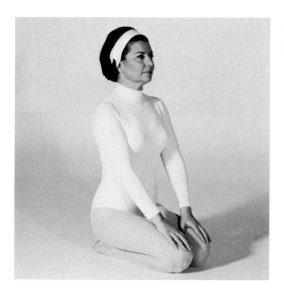

Kneel with legs tucked under buttocks. Rest hands on knees and sit up so that spine is perfectly straight, but not rigid.

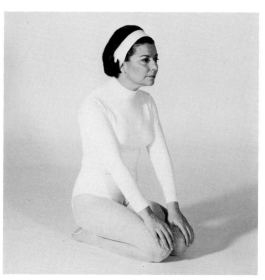

To tone throat and chin line, stretch neck as far out as you can without moving shoulders. You should feel the pull in your throat, chin line and back of neck. Hold tautly for 5 seconds. Repeat three times.

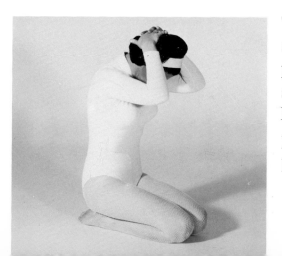

To loosen tight muscles in back of neck and shoulders, clasp hands behind head and pull downward, using resistance to feel stretch along back of neck. Hold 5 seconds. Repeat three times.

For additional head and neck exercises see Exercises 60 and 68.

13. FIRMING UNDERSIDES OF ARMS AND IMPROVING POSTURE

In addition to firming the undersides of the arms and improving the posture, you exercise the lungs, too, when deep breathing is synchronized with these movements.

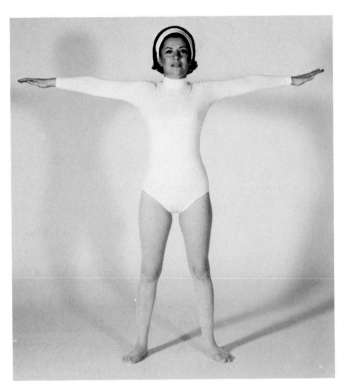

Stand with feet apart, arms outstretched at sides. Inhale deeply while stretching arms as far out as possible without tensing neck. You should feel pull on undersides of arms and in the shoulders and back. Hold the pose and breath for 5 seconds. Exhale. Repeat three times.

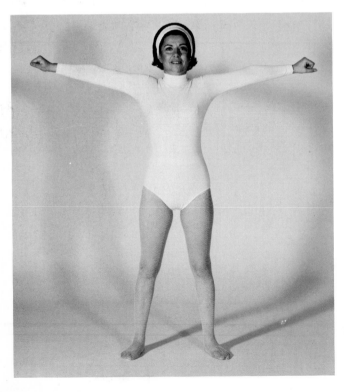

In the same position, outstretch arms with fists clenched. Rotate arms five times in a forward motion while drawing in a long, uninterrupted breath. Exhale. Repeat three times.

For additional arm-firming and posture exercises see Exercises 66 and 70.

14. BALANCING EXERCISES

Balance, posture and concentration are emphasized in the Vertical Stretch and Knee Bend. To maintain better balance, concentrate on an object at eye level. It can be a picture, a lamp or any object close enough for focus.

At first you may need the use of a support—a table or chair—but you will soon find your point of balance and control.

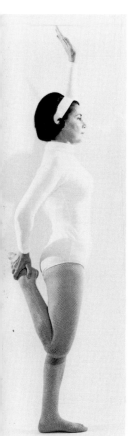

Vertical Stretch:
Stand firmly on left leg, putting full weight on it. Bend right leg behind, grasping the foot with right hand. Steady balance while concentrating on an object at eye level. Inhale and at the same time lift left arm, fingers pointing upward. While breathing freely, stretch to feel pull in the spine. Hold for 10–15 seconds. Relax.
Stand on right leg and repeat same movements. Repeat four times, alternating the left and right legs.

Knee Bend:
Stand firmly on left leg to steady your balance. Bend right knee in front as high as possible. Clasp leg below knee with both hands. Inhale. Pull knee in toward chest, toes down. Breathe freely and stretch spine upward for about 10–15 seconds. Concentrate on an object at eye level to steady your balance. Exhale, lower leg, and relax. Stand on right leg, bend left knee and repeat same movements. Repeat four times, alternating the left and right legs. Relax completely.

This is the last exercise of the second stage. While relaxing, do a little deep breathing before concluding the session.

As you become more deeply involved in yoga, greater demands will be made on your power of concentration and in further stretching, limbering and toning exercises.

"Infinite energy," says writer Adams Beck, "is at the disposal of man if he knows how to get it, and this is a part of the science of yoga."

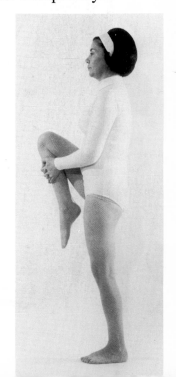

Summary of the Third Stage

Exercise Time: 10 Minutes

BENEFITS

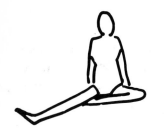 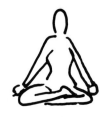 PERFECT POSTURE	Develops flexibility in hips, knees and ankles; frees legs and weight of body from muscular tension; has calming effect on nervous system.
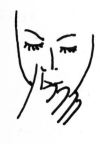 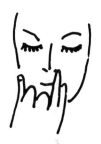 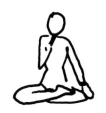 ALTERNATE BREATHING	Cleanses nasal passages; calms the mind; especially helpful in preventing buildup of tension; helps to relieve sinus headache.
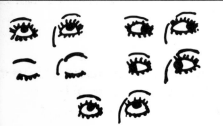 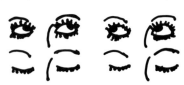 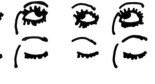 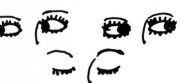 EYE EXERCISES	Reduces fatigue and eyestrain; strengthens optic nerves and muscles.
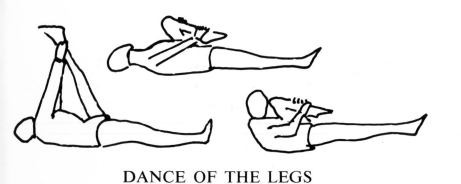 DANCE OF THE LEGS	Firms abdomen, buttocks, and thighs; all-around toning and limbering exercise.

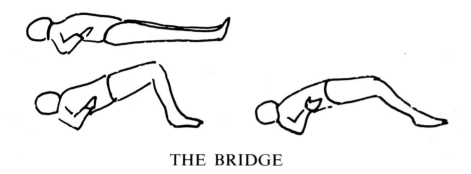

THE BRIDGE

Strengthens weak muscles of lumbar region; increases suppleness of spine; strengthens arms and wrists.

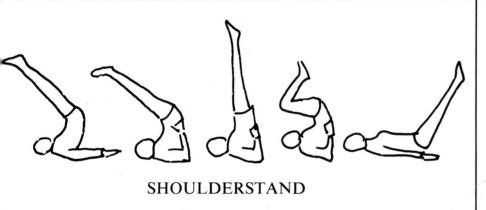

SHOULDERSTAND

Restores youth and vitality; tones endocrine glands; delays aging process; improves circulation; relieves varicose veins; reduces swollen feet and ankles; relief for sinus sufferers. Excellent beauty treatment; stimulates and tones facial muscles.

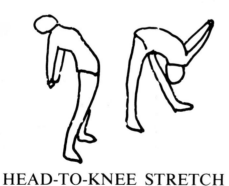

HEAD-TO-KNEE STRETCH

Corrects round shoulders and poor posture; limbers all muscles of body; exercises lungs through deep breathing.

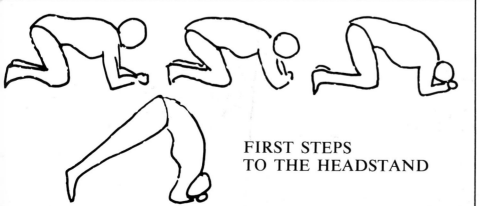

FIRST STEPS TO THE HEADSTAND

Strengthens neck and back muscles; firms legs; sends fresh supply of blood to brain.

15. PERFECT POSTURE

When first practicing the Perfect Posture, you may find it more comfortable to sit on a small cushion that will slightly raise your body and lower your legs. Your knees may stubbornly rest in the air, but with practice they will gradually limber. *Don't force your legs into this position.* If your knees are stiff, simply sit in the Easy Posture, shown in Exercise 8, to practice the breathing.

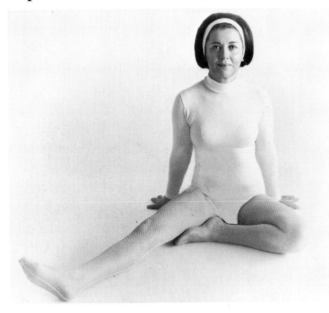

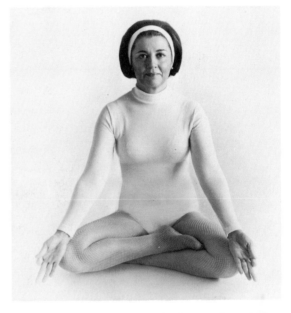

Sit with legs apart, spine straight, hands to sides of body. Bend left leg so that sole of foot rests against inner right thigh close to the crotch.

Place right leg over left so that foot rests against left inner thigh and ankles meet, right over left. Rest hands on knees, palms up. Fingers form the "Symbol of Knowledge" pose: thumb and index finger make a circle, and the middle, ring and little fingers are extended. Close your eyes and hold this pose for about 20 seconds while breathing deeply and calmly. Focus your mind on the rhythm of the breath. Then relax your legs and bounce them up and down a few times to stimulate circulation. Reverse the position, crossing left leg over the right, and repeat deep breathing.

16. HEAD-TO-KNEE STRETCH

These forward and backward stretches not only help to limber the spine but will correct round shoulders and a poor posture. The lungs too are thoroughly exercised through the deep-breathing movements.

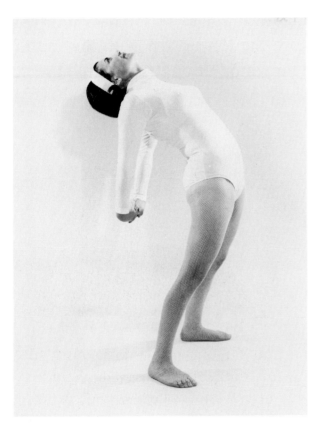

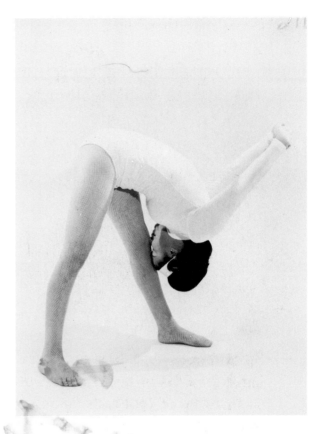

Stand with feet apart, hands clasped behind, eyes closed. Inhale while bending backward to arch neck and spine. Stretch clasped hands back and out.

Exhale while slowly bending forward until head touches left knee, or as far as possible. Arms are stretched back and up. Breathe freely for 5 seconds while holding the pose to benefit from the stretch. Inhale, and at the same time slowly come up; bend backward once more, arching neck and spine. Hold the breath and stretch arms out and back. Exhale and return to standing position. Repeat four times, alternating the right and left legs.

17. ALTERNATE BREATHING

To become familiar with this breathing pattern, read the instructions first before closing your eyes to let your mind take quiet control over the breath. The rhythm should be deep and smooth, the breath flowing into and out of the nostrils alternately.

If your nose is blocked and breathing becomes difficult, press your right thumb on the right nostril and forcefully inhale and exhale through the left nostril 15 to 20 times. Then close the left nostril with the fourth finger and repeat the same deep forceful breathing through the right nostril. This should ease your breathing considerably.

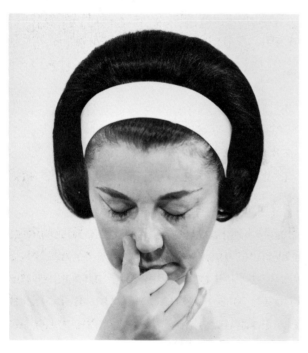 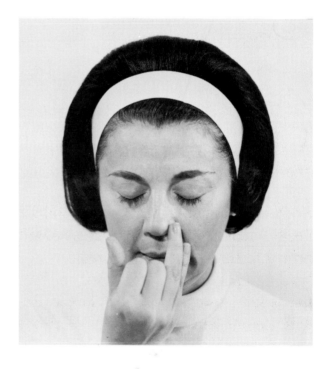

Position of Right Hand:
Bend index and middle fingers toward palm. Place right hand close to the nose with thumb near the right nostril. When inhaling, press thumb on nostril and breathe in through left nostril.

When exhaling, press fourth finger on left nostril, release thumb, and breathe out through right nostril.

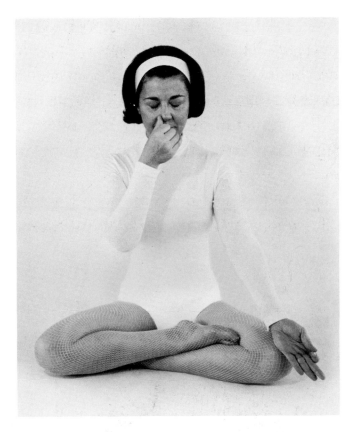

Position of Left Hand:
Sit in one of the meditative postures.
Outstretch left arm, palm up and
resting on knee. Fingers form the
"Symbol of Knowledge" pose.

Alternate Breathing Pattern:

Press right thumb on right nostril. Inhale
deeply and smoothly through the left
nostril to the count of 5 seconds.

Close left nostril with fourth finger. Release thumb and slowly exhale through
the right nostril to the count of 10
seconds.

Without releasing finger from left nostril,
inhale through the right to the count of
5 seconds.

Close right nostril with thumb, at the
same time releasing left nostril, and
exhale to the count of 10 seconds.

This is one round of Alternate Breathing.
Practice until you are able to do three
rounds without stopping, allowing the
breath to flow steadily into and out of
the nostrils. Then increase the ratio for
each round as follows:

Inhale to the count of	6	seconds
Exhale "	12	"
Inhale "	7	"
Exhale "	14	"
Inhale "	8	"
Exhale "	16	"

18. EYE EXERCISES

These slow and deliberate eye movements are done either sitting or lying flat *without moving the head.* Glasses should be removed during the exercises. Imagine that you are "dragging" your muscles in the different movements to feel the pull. Repeat each exercise three times and hold about three seconds. Close your eyes, rest a second, then proceed with the next movement.

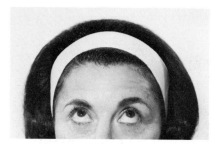 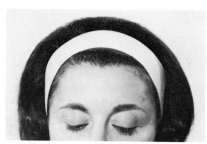

Eyes up, eyes down.

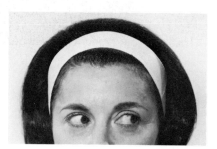 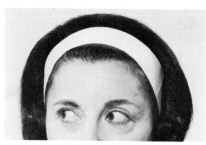

Eyes left, eyes right.

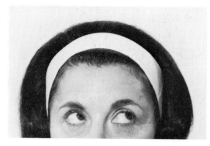 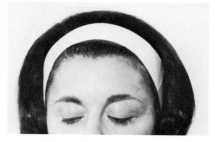

Eyes upper left, eyes lower right.

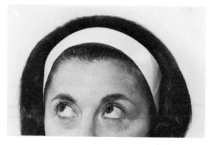 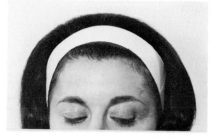

Eyes upper right, eyes lower left.

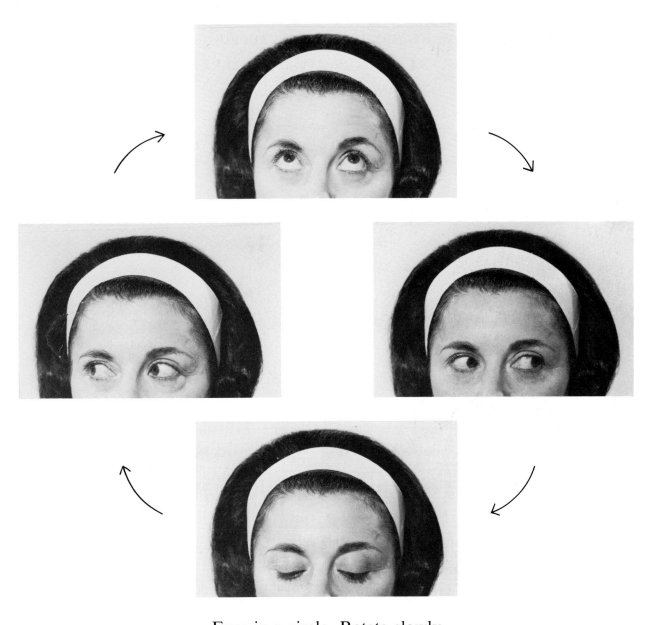

Eyes in a circle. Rotate slowly
three times without stopping:
up, left, down and right. Reverse rotation.

Changing Focus: This eye exercise will be helpful
during any sustained close work. Change your
focus by moving your eyes from a distant point to
a closer one. Repeat ten times, slowly shifting the
focus back and forth.

19. DANCE OF THE LEGS

The rhythmic movements of this exercise give the body an all-around toning and limbering effect, and will help firm the abdomen, buttocks and thighs.

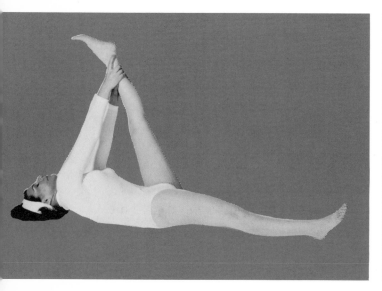 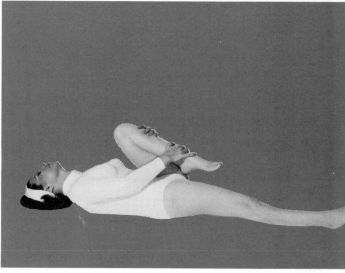

20. THE BRIDGE

Here is a good exercise to strengthen weak muscles of the lumbar region—frequently the cause of back ailments. The Bridge also adds suppleness to the spine and strengthens arms and wrists.

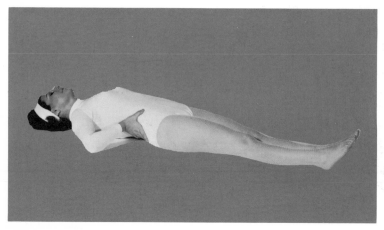 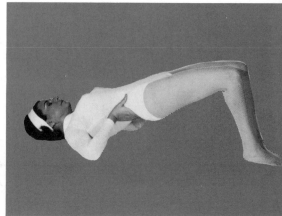

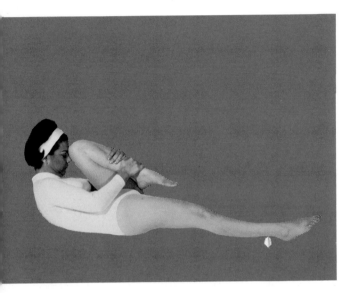

Lie flat on back, arms overhead, eyes closed. Inhale while raising left leg straight and as high as possible. At the same time bring arms up to grasp left ankle (or as far as you can reach without straining). Right leg remains on floor.

Exhale, tightening abdomen while still grasping left leg. Bend the leg and bring close to chest.

Raise head to meet knee. Breathe freely and hold pose for 5 seconds. Inhale while slowly lowering head with arms returning to overhead position
and leg returning to the floor. Exhale.

Repeat with right leg. Then repeat same movements raising both legs.

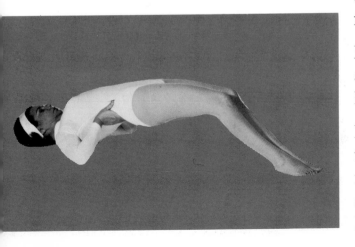

Lie flat on your back. Grasp waist with thumbs up, elbows bent and resting on the floor.

Inhale while bending knees. With help of arms, arch spine as high as possible; keep head on floor without straining the neck.

Breathe freely as you slide the feet forward to create a wide bridge between head and feet. Hold the pose and your breath for 5 seconds. Inhale as you lower the spine and legs. Exhale. Repeat three times.

21. THE SHOULDERSTAND

The Shoulderstand is a restorer of youth and vitality. It is one yoga posture most people are able to do, some more easily than others. If your back muscles are weak, you may have a little difficulty raising your legs. In that case roll back, using a little momentum so that you can raise your hips.

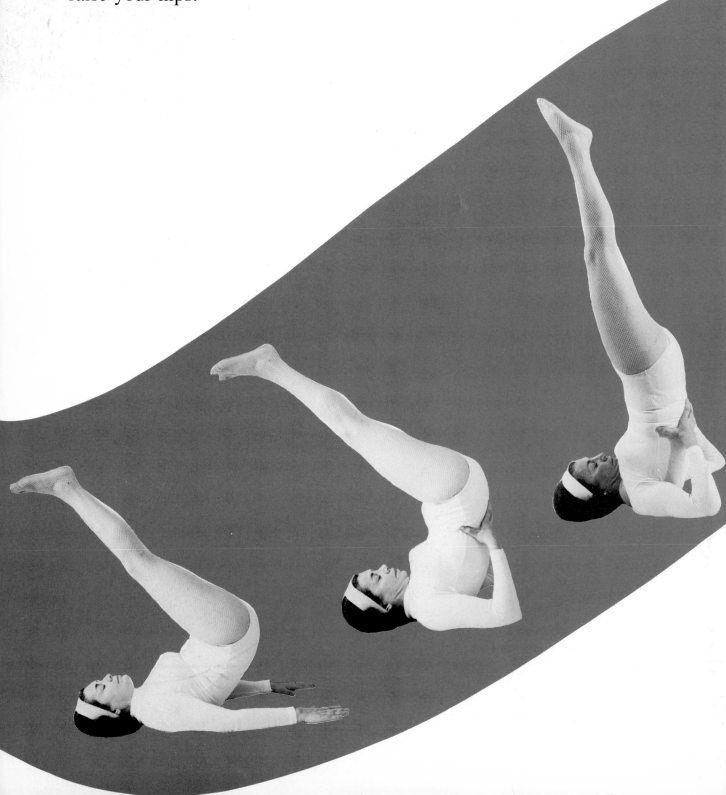

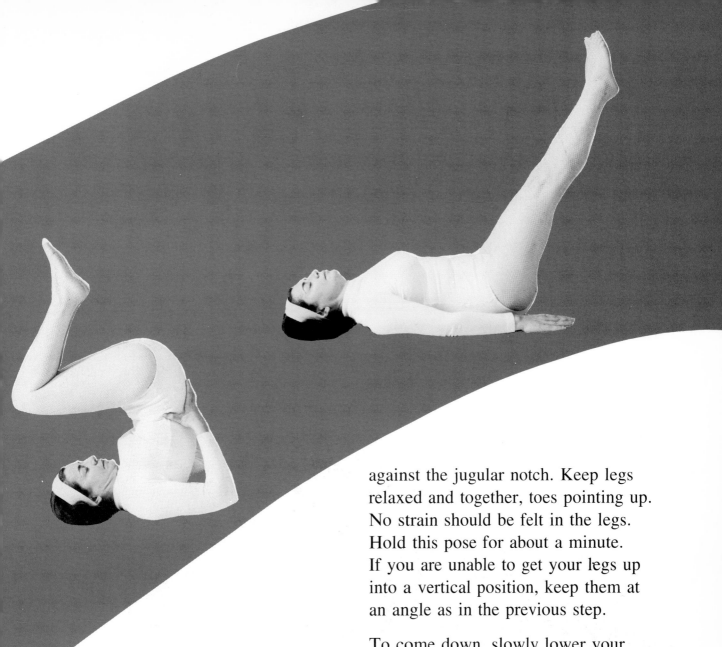

Lie flat on your back, legs together, palms down close to sides. Close your eyes. Inhale as you raise legs over your head, knees straight, or roll back.

Support your back with hands. Breathe freely.

Continue to raise your legs by pushing the hips with your hands until legs are in a vertical position. Weight of body should be on the shoulders and arms, with chin pressing against the jugular notch. Keep legs relaxed and together, toes pointing up. No strain should be felt in the legs. Hold this pose for about a minute. If you are unable to get your legs up into a vertical position, keep them at an angle as in the previous step.

To come down, slowly lower your legs by bending the knees. (You can eliminate this step if you are able to lower your legs without bending them.)

Let your hands slip farther down along the hips till your back is on the floor with palms down. If you arch your neck back as you straighten your legs, you will be able to keep your head on the floor. As much as possible use abdominal muscles when lowering the legs to free the shoulders from muscular tension.
Repeat twice.

49

22. FIRST STEPS TO THE HEADSTAND

Even if you have no intention of standing on your head, these preliminary steps to the Headstand will strengthen neck and lumbar muscles, and also firm the legs. When the head is lowered in reverse position, a fresh supply of blood is sent to the brain.

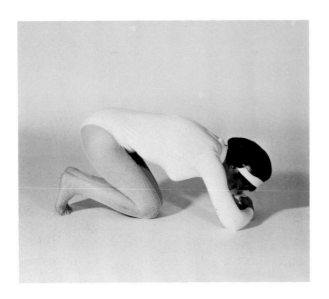

Kneel with legs together, body forward, head lowered with arms in front. To measure the right distance for your arms, bend each arm so that fingertips touch the elbow of other arm.

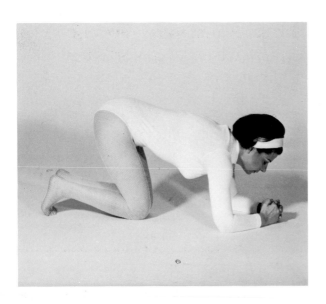

Without moving the elbows, stretch out arms and interlock the fingers. You now have the correct distance.

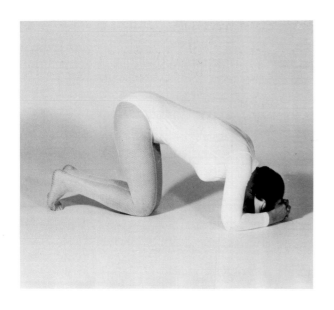

Bend head down with top of head resting on the floor. Place clasped hands to encircle head. The neck and head must feel comfortable, so find your own point of balance.

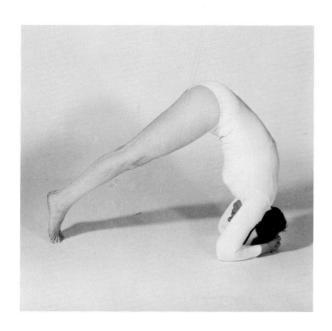

Straighten legs by unbending the knees and resting on your toes. Take a few steps "walking in" toward your head, then a few steps back. Repeat five times. Then rock back and forth ten times on your toes by raising and lowering the heels. Bend knees and slowly come out of the Headstand position. Repeat twice. (See first step of Exercise 43 for "walking in" practice.)

Lie on your back and relax completely while breathing deeply for a few extra minutes before concluding this third stage. When practicing yoga, remember to keep the pace slow and rhythmic to gain maximum benefit. Frequent rests are important.

Summary of the Fourth Stage

Exercise Time: 10 Minutes

BENEFITS

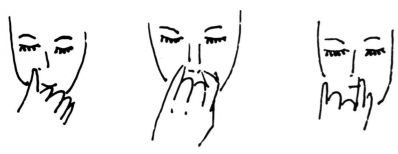

ALTERNATE BREATHING WITH RETENTION

Inhalation: lungs and cells are filled with air.

Retention: Exchange of gaseous substance. Toxic air is replaced by fresh air in the tissues and lungs.

Exhalation: All toxic air is removed from lungs.

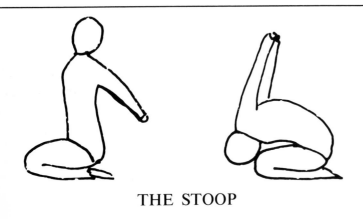

THE STOOP

Massages and tones entire abdominal and pelvic area; helps to correct irregular elimination; firms hips; limbers knees and ankles; improves posture; exercises lungs.

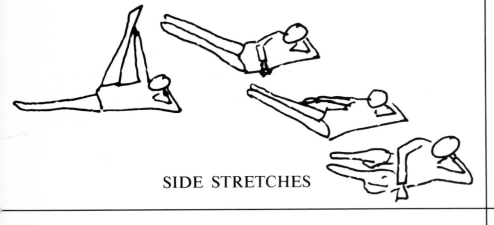

SIDE STRETCHES

Improves balance; slims waistline, hips and thighs.

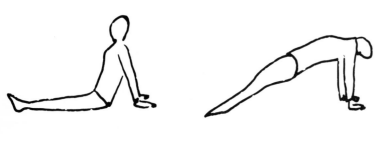

THE INCLINED PLANE

Stretches pelvis; strengthens and firms arms, hips, back and thighs.

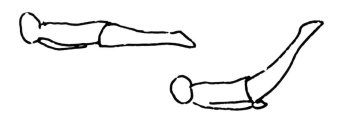

THE LOCUST

Tones muscles of abdomen and lower back; firms buttocks, hips and thighs; brings rich supply of blood to brain.

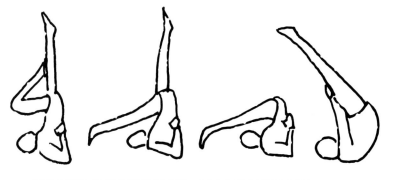

SPINAL TWIST

Brings about strong cross pull of spinal column; increases elasticity of spine; slims waistline; releases tension in back muscles; improves posture.

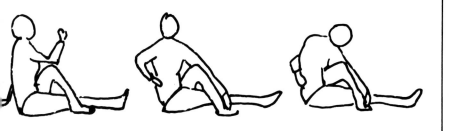

SHOULDERSTAND VARIATIONS

Restores elasticity to spine; limbers and tones legs; improves circulation with calming effect on entire body and mind; tones facial muscles.

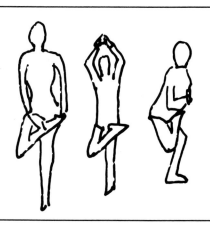

THE TREE

Improves balance by power of concentration; limbers legs; improves posture.

23. ALTERNATE BREATHING WITH RETENTION

Sit in a meditative pose, either the Easy or the Perfect posture. You may also sit in a chair if these positions are uncomfortable.

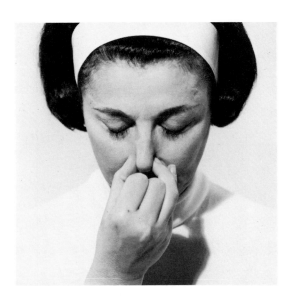

Press right thumb on right nostril. Inhale deeply and smoothly through the left to the count of 5 seconds.

Close left nostril without releasing right. Retain breath to the count of 20 seconds.

Release right nostril and exhale to the count of 10 seconds.

Inhale through right nostril to the count of 5 seconds. Close it without releasing left nostril. Retain breath to the count of 20 seconds.

Release left nostril and exhale to the count of 10 seconds.

This is one round of Alternate Breathing with Retention. Repeat two rounds without stopping.

Your breath should be so well controlled that no tension is felt in the body. Gradually increase the breathing pattern to these ratios:

Inhale	6 seconds	Inhale	7 seconds
Retain	24 "	Retain	28 "
Exhale	12 "	Exhale	14 "

When you have acquired full control of the 7:28:14 ratio, then increase the breathing to three rounds without stopping. Begin with 5:20:10, proceed to 6:24:12, and the last round will be 7:28:14.

24. THE STOOP

This posture is a simplified version of the traditional *Yoga Mudra* shown in Exercise 46, done in the Lotus position. Fingers remain interlocked throughout the movements.

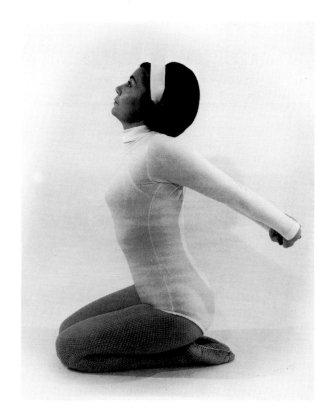

Kneel with legs tucked under the buttocks (or sit in the Lotus pose), spine straight, fingers interlocked behind back. Inhale deeply while stretching arms back and out, keeping spine straight.

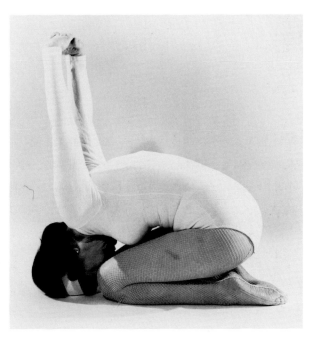

Exhale while bending forward and down with arms straight up, fingers interlocked, until head touches the floor without raising hips. Stretch should be felt in the spine and arms. Breathe freely and hold pose for 5 seconds, at the same time pulling in the abdomen. Inhale, slowly come up to kneeling position, exhale. Repeat twice.

25. SIDE STRETCHES

This sequence of side stretches, which does wonders for the waistline, hips and thighs and improves balance, should be repeated four times: twice on the left side and twice on the right. For maximum benefit, hold each pose for 5 seconds while breathing freely.

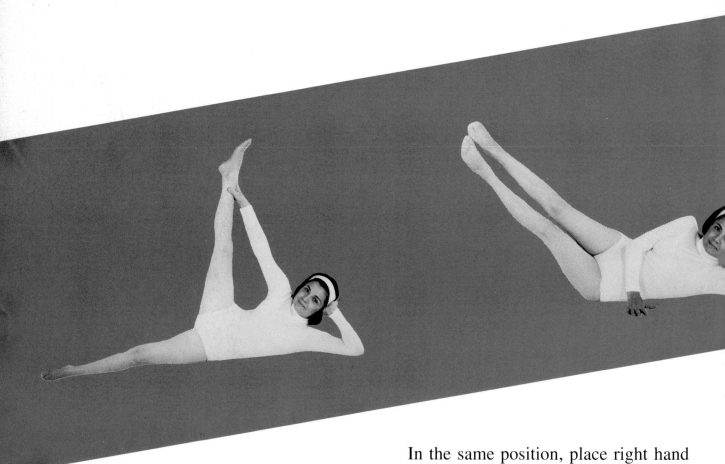

Lie on your left side, left elbow bent with hand resting to support head. Right hand is outstretched on thigh. Inhale and raise right leg high, keeping knee straight. Grasp ankle. Breathe freely and hold pose, then release ankle and lower leg.

In the same position, place right hand on the floor, palm down close to chest. Inhale. Raise both legs up without bending knees. Breathe freely and hold pose, then lower legs.

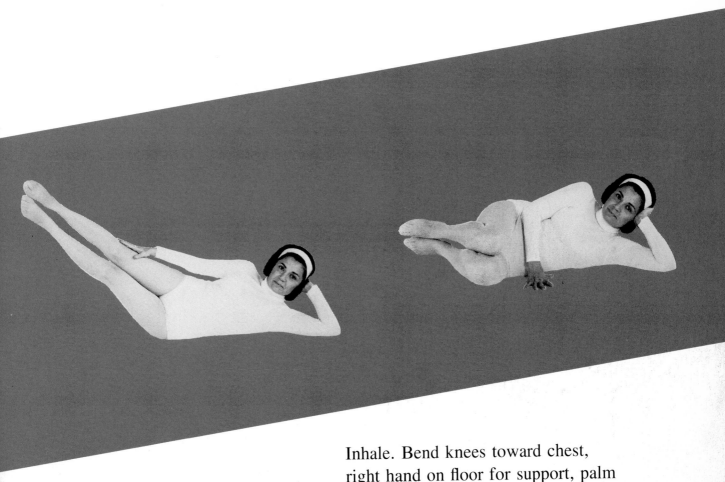

Repeat last exercise, but balance without support of right hand. Place it along the right side while raising legs. Breathe freely and hold pose, then lower legs.

Inhale. Bend knees toward chest, right hand on floor for support, palm pressing down. Breathe freely. Without touching floor straighten legs, then bend them again toward the chest. Repeat 5 times without stopping. Lower legs and relax.

26. THE INCLINED PLANE

When the body is on an inclined plane there should be no sag in the middle, so that the pelvis can be stretched and the arms, hips, back and thighs strengthened and firmed.

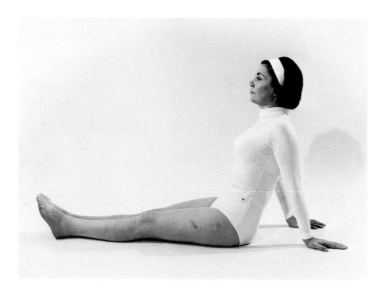

Sit with legs outstretched and together, arms behind with palms resting flat, fingers pointing away from body.

With eyes closed, inhale and raise torso. Weight should rest entirely on palms and feet (or heels if you cannot reach that far). While breathing freely, hold pose for 5 seconds. Then lower torso to sitting position with arms behind as before. Repeat three times.

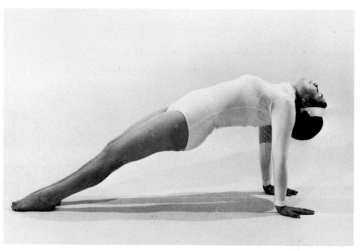

A variation of this posture is shown in Exercise 48.

27. THE LOCUST

This posture helps to tone muscles of the abdomen and lower back while firming the buttocks, hips and thighs. Holding the legs suspended for 5 seconds will make you feel the blood rush to your face. This is a good beauty treatment.

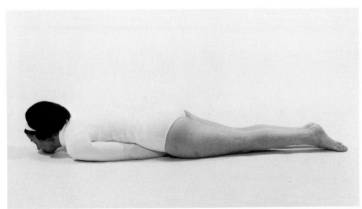

Lie face down, chin on floor, nose up, legs together, eyes closed. Clench fist and place them close together, thumbs touching, under the groin.

Inhale deeply. Press fist against floor to thrust legs upward as high as possible keeping head down, knees straight. Hold pose for 5 seconds. If possible, hold your breath for this period; otherwise, breathe freely. Exhale; lower legs. Repeat three times.

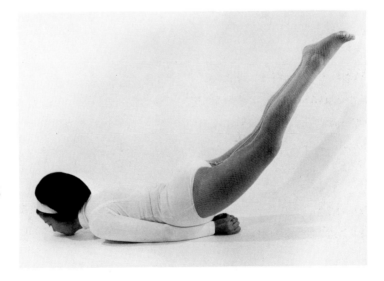

28. SHOULDERSTAND VARIATIONS

By now your muscular control in the Shoulderstand should be sufficiently developed to enable you to do these variations for further limbering and toning.

Each exercise should be done twice without lowering the body, and the pose held for 5 seconds while breathing freely.

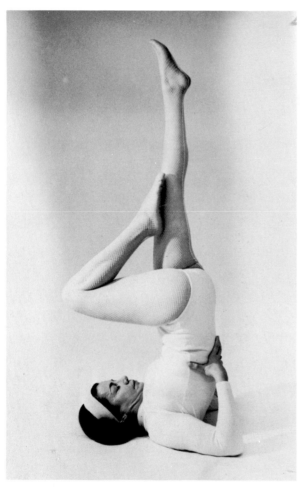

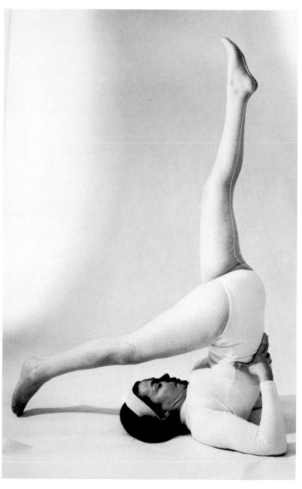

With legs in the Shoulderstand pose (Exercise 21, Step 3), inhale and bend right knee with sole of foot close to left knee. Chin is pressed against jugular notch. Hold the pose; then straighten right leg to vertical position. Repeat with left leg.

Inhale and lower right leg over head without bending the knee until toes touch floor (or as far down as you can reach). Hold the pose, then return leg to vertical position.
Repeat with left leg.

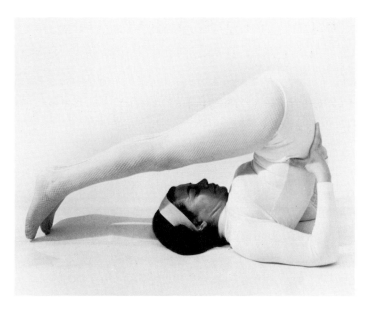

Inhale and lower both legs over head without bending knees until toes touch the floor (or as far down as you can reach). Hold pose while pulling in abdominal muscles. Then return to vertical position.

Inhale and lower legs a little over head without bending knees. Elbows support body with hands gripping waist. When balance is secure, slowly remove hands and place them on the thighs. Balance in this "pose of tranquillity." Return to vertical position with hands supporting body, then gradually lower legs to the floor.

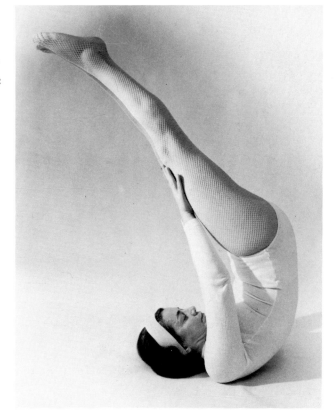

For additional Shoulderstand variations see Exercise 47.

29. SPINAL TWIST

At first glance this posture looks tricky; it is more easily done than explained. You should have no difficulty if you can remember that the right hand crosses over the left leg, and vice versa.

It is one of the best yoga exercises to release tension in back muscles and increase the spine's elasticity, as well as slim the waistline.

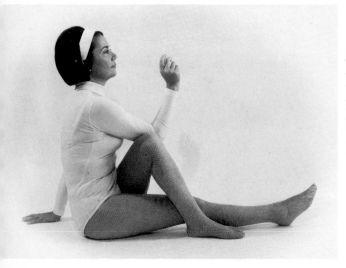

Sit with legs outstretched and together. Bend left knee and cross left leg over right. Left foot should touch right knee. Right elbow is bent and rests on outer side of left knee. Left hand is stretched back, palm flat on floor.

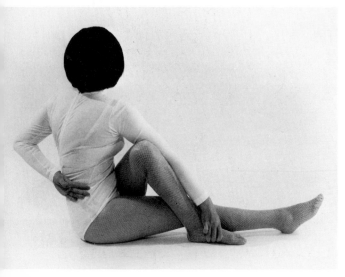

Now stretch right hand to grasp the left foot, with elbow touching left knee. (If you are unable to do this, then encircle your right arm around the left knee, bringing it close to your chest.) Now place left hand behind back with back of hand touching spine. Inhale. Look up over your left shoulder, eyes toward the ceiling. Hold your breath and the pose for 5 seconds.

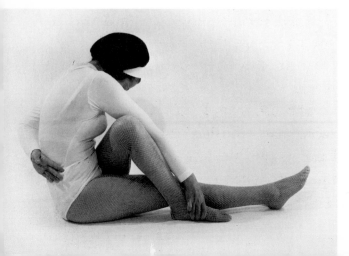

Exhale as you turn your head forward and down to relax. Repeat twice: inhale, look up, exhale, head down. Then repeat same movements crossing the right leg over the left with left hand grasping right foot.

This posture is called the Half–Spinal Twist. The Full Spinal Twist is shown in Exercise 49.

30. THE TREE

This symbolic posture of a tree is an exercise of balance, posture and concentration. Focus on an object at eye level to steady your balance.

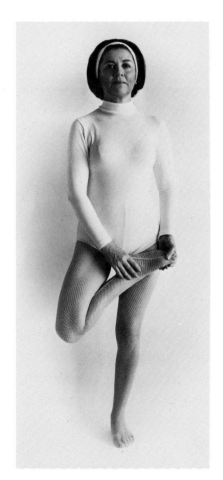 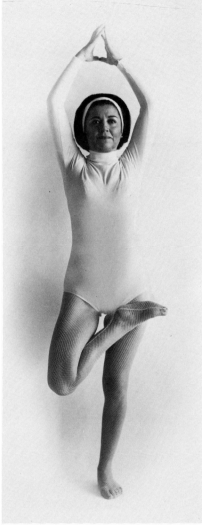 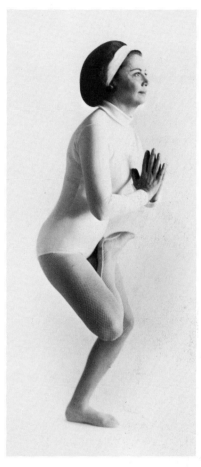

Stand firmly on left leg. Bring right leg up over left thigh, sole of foot facing up. Grasp foot and ankle with both hands and press foot against thigh. Inhale and slowly raise arms overhead, fingertips touching. Breathe freely while concentrating on the tree image. Then bend left knee a little and bring palms close to chest, keeping head and spine in a line. Hold for 10–15 seconds.
Repeat with right leg, bringing left leg over right thigh. Repeat four times, alternating the left and right legs. If this exercise is too difficult, try the simplified version of The Tree in Exercise 94.

Relax completely for a few minutes while breathing deeply. Think about the spirit of yoga and what it can do for you.

The *Bhagavad Gita* says that "the wise man who has conquered his mind and is absorbed in the Self is as a lamp which does not flicker, since it stands sheltered from every wind."

Summary of the Fifth Stage
Exercise Time: 10 Minutes

BENEFITS

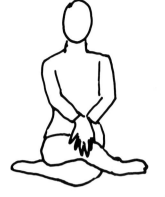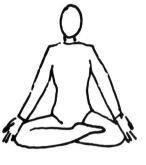

Hero Posture   Half-Lotus Posture
MEDITATIVE SITTING POSTURES

Both postures increase flexibility of legs.

RHYTHMIC VIBRATIONS OF SOUNDS:
> Hissing Breath
> Droning Breath

Creates subtle sound vibrations for calming influence on mind.

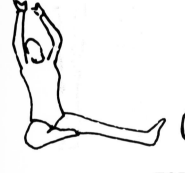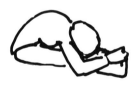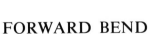

FORWARD BEND

Gives body a vigorous toning up; stretches all muscles, particularly those of hips, legs and pelvis; makes spine more elastic.

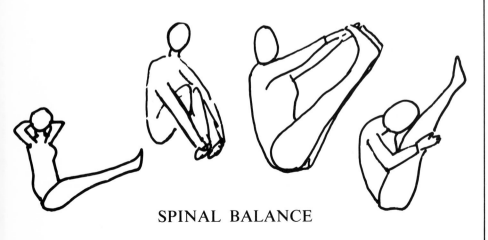

SPINAL BALANCE

Strengthens abdominal muscles; firms hips, buttocks and legs.

64

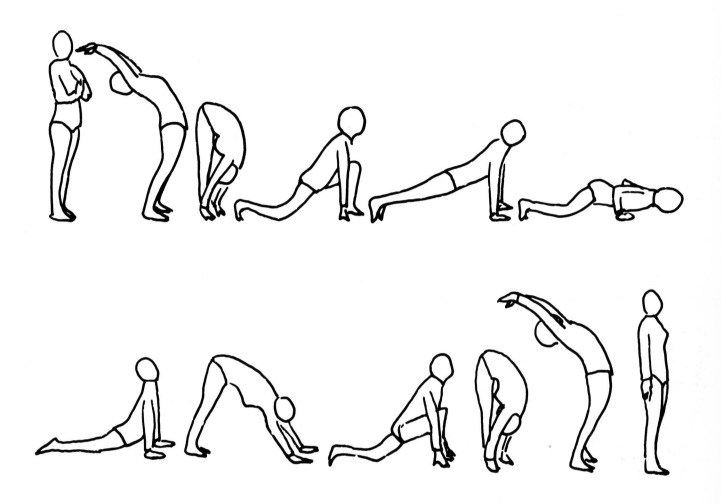

SUN SALUTATION

BENEFITS

Spinal movements stretch various
ligaments and muscles to increase
elasticity of the vertebral column
and joints. Excellent warm-up for
early-morning exercise.

31. THE HERO POSTURE

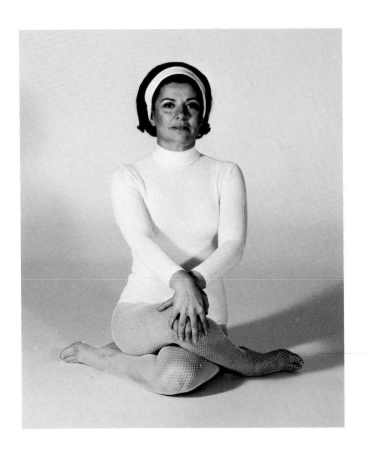

Sit with legs outstretched, hands to sides. Bend left leg so that heel rests beside right thigh. Bend right leg over the left with knees in line. Right heel is close to left thigh. Place left palm with right over it on the knee. Fingers are interlaced. Keep spine straight with head in line. Close your eyes and breathe deeply for a few seconds to distract the mind from the new stretch in the legs.

Repeat the same movements with left leg over the right, and left palm over the right. Then stretch your legs; bounce them up and down to stimulate circulation.

32. HALF-LOTUS POSTURE

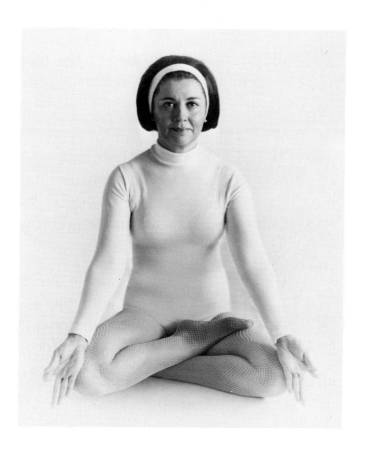

Sit with legs outstretched and apart, hands to sides. Spine, head and shoulders are held in perfect alignment, ribs are lifted, abdomen held in.

Bend left leg so heel is close to inner right thigh. Bend right leg over left, bringing foot close to the crotch or wherever it will be comfortable without straining the leg. Rest hands on knees in the "Symbol of Knowledge" pose. Close your eyes and breathe deeply for a few seconds so that your body will become accustomed to the new stretch.

Relax your legs. Repeat the same movements reversing the left leg over the right.

A variation of the Half-Lotus is shown in Exercise 50.

33. RHYTHMIC VIBRATIONS OF SOUND
DRONING AND HISSING BREATHS

Subtle sound vibrations created through the Droning and Hissing Breaths can have a calming influence on the mind when done with maximum power of concentration and strong breath control.

Sit in one of the meditative postures for these breathing exercises.

THE DRONING BREATH:

When the breath is slowly released with controlled humming it is similar to the sound of a droning bee. Resonance is felt in the upper nasal passages between the eyebrows. This is where the point of concentration lies.

To the count of 8 seconds, inhale deeply and forcibly through the nose. Then with lips slightly parted, hum as you exhale, slowly and forcibly, to the count of 16 seconds. Repeat three times without stopping.

THE HISSING BREATH:

This is also an exercise to control the outgoing breath. Lips are pressed against the teeth while the breath is released in a slow and controlled hissing sound. Point of concentration is between the eyebrows.

To the count of 8 seconds, inhale deeply and forcibly through the nose. With lips pressed against the teeth, release the breath slowly and evenly in a strong hissing sound to the count of 16 seconds. Repeat three times without stopping.

34. FORWARD BEND

Most of the muscles are stretched in these forward bends, particularly those of the hips, legs and pelvis, which get a vigorous toning up.

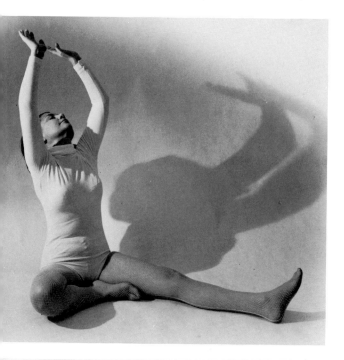

1.

Sit with legs apart. Bend right leg so that foot rests close to inner left thigh. Inhale; raise arms, stretching upward.

2.

Exhale; bend forward with head touching left knee (or as far forward as you can reach). Breathe freely and grasp left foot with both hands. If possible, bend elbows for a greater stretch. Hold pose for 10 seconds. Then inhale; slowly sit up with arms overhead as before. Exhale; lower arms to the sides. Repeat with left leg.

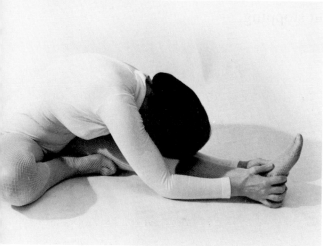

3.

Sit with legs together. Inhale; raise arms, stretching upward. Exhale; bend forward with head touching the knees (or as far down as you can reach). Breathing freely, grasp the big toes, with elbows touching the floor—if possible. Hold the pose for 10 seconds to feel the stretch in the legs, arms and spine. Then inhale; slowly sit up with arms overhead. Exhale; lower arms to the sides. Repeat twice.

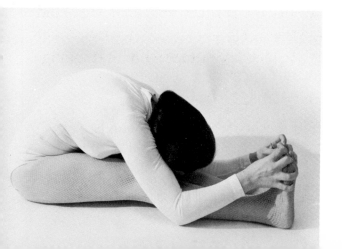

35. SPINAL BALANCE

In this Spinal Balance sequence, abdominal muscles are strengthened, hips and legs are firmed. Each exercise should be done twice, and the pose held for 10–15 seconds.

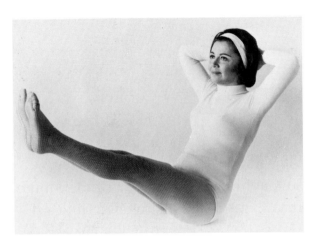

Clasp hands behind head. Inhale; bend slightly back to raise legs with knees straight. Hold the pose, then relax.

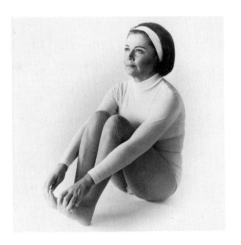

Bend knees close to body and grip toes.

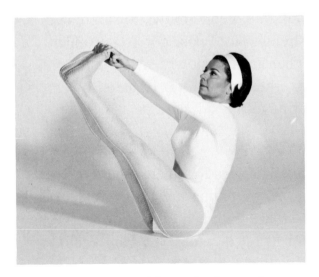

Then raise legs without losing grip on toes. (If this is too difficult, balance against a wall and try to raise one leg at a time.)

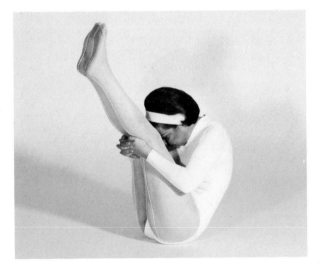

When balance is secure, bend head close to knees and clasp hands behind knees.

Hold the pose, then relax hands and place palms flat on floor while lowering legs.

36. SUN SALUTATION

At first glance, this series of twelve postures seems confusing. If you practice them individually, you will be able to memorize the movements so that they will flow together in a continuous rhythmic motion with synchronized breathing. You will notice that posture 11 is the same as posture 2. In posture 4 the left leg is brought forward, while in posture 9 the right leg comes forward. The breathing is easy to remember: inhale as you bend back, exhale as you bend forward. Retain your breath in posture 5. Each posture should be held for about 3 seconds. To increase the stretch in the spine, when moving from one posture into the next keep palms in the same position, without shifting.

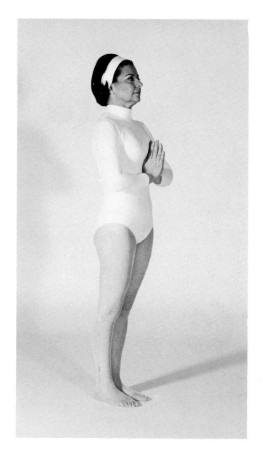

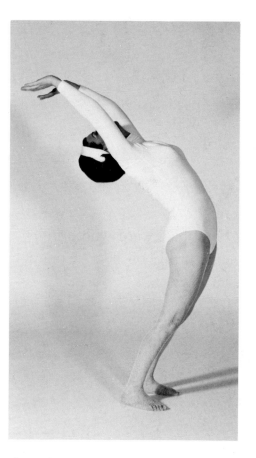

1. Stand erect with legs together, palms touching close to chest.

2. Inhale; raise arms overhead. Bend back to arch spine.

Continued ▶

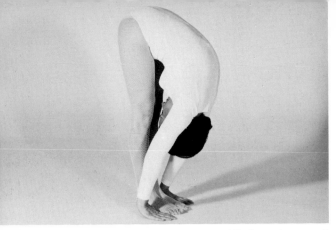

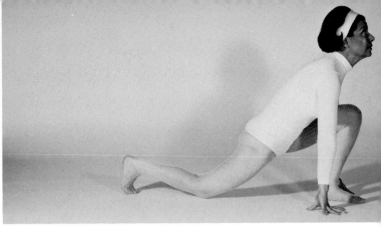

3. Exhale; bend forward till hands are in line with feet. Contract abdomen and bring head close to knees. Knees are kept straight.

4. Inhale; move right leg in a backward step, knee touching floor. Keep left foot firmly on floor; left knee is between hands. (When repeating exercise, reverse position of legs.)

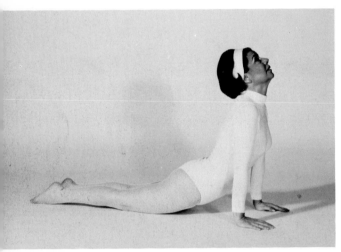

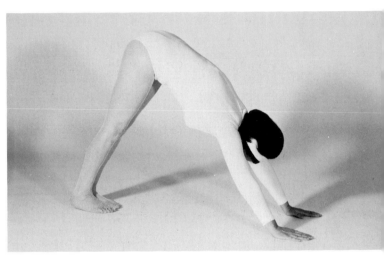

7. Inhale; bend backward with arms straight, palms firmly on floor. Contract back muscles.

8. Exhale; arch back in a cat's stretch, head down between arms. Do not strain; keep head limp.

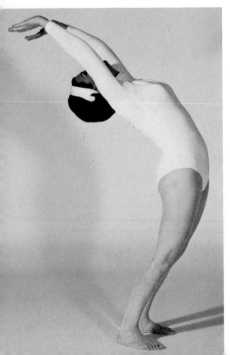

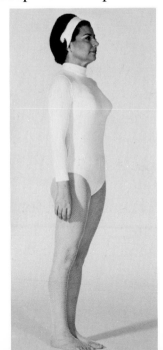

11. Inhale; raise arms overhead. Bend back to arch spine.

12. Exhale; lower arms to the sides.

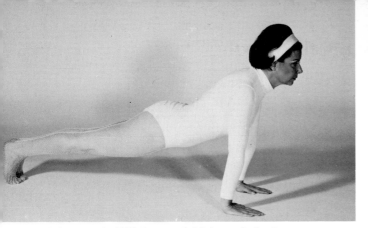

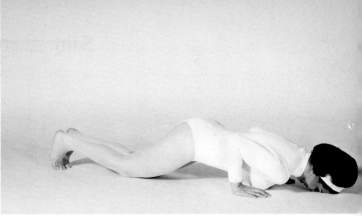

5. Hold breath. Without shifting right leg, raise knee off the floor, then move left leg, in a backward step to meet right foot. Toes are turned in and body is elevated on an even plane with arms fully stretched and palms firmly on floor. Look straight ahead.

6. Exhale; bend knees to touch floor without shifting palms. Then lower body so that forehead and chest come in contact with the floor. In this position your buttocks, chin and nose are off the floor.

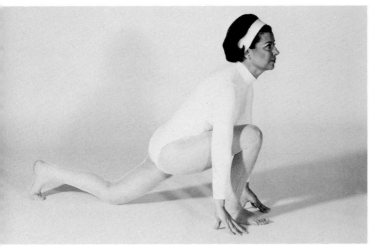

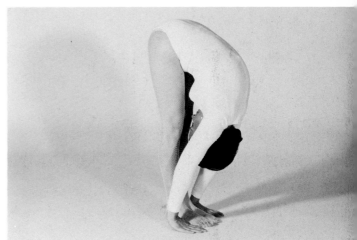

9. Inhale; bring right leg forward alongside palms. Left foot and knee touch floor. (When repeating exercise, reverse position of legs.)

10. Exhale; bend forward till hands are in line with feet, palms flat on floor. Contract abdomen and bring head close to knees. Knees are straight.

Repeat Sun Salutation twice. As your stamina and flexibility increase, you will enjoy doing this exercise three to four times as a warm-up to loosen tight muscles and give your body greater freedom of movement. Start slowly, holding each posture for 3 seconds. Then 2 seconds for the second time, 1 second for the third time, and half a second for the fourth time. By the end of the fourth time, the movements should be swift and rhythmic.

Rest completely after the Sun Salutation. This is the end of the Fifth Stage. Breathe deeply to enjoy a mental state of repose.

"When the mind gains peace, right discrimination follows," says the *Bhagavad Gita.*

Summary of the Sixth Stage

Exercise Time: 10 Minutes

	BENEFITS
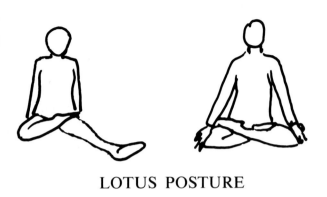 **LOTUS POSTURE**	Gives legs, hips and pelvis greater flexibility; corrects slouching when legs are locked in Lotus pose.
BELLOWS BREATH	Recharges breath as lungs, diaphragm and abdominal muscles are exerted to utmost while body remains still; tones up nervous system; restores vitality; has exhilarating effect on mind and body.
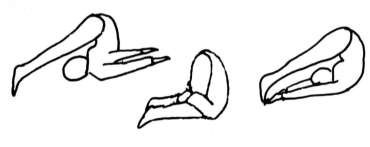 **THE PLOW AND VARIATIONS**	Massages liver and spleen; limbers each vertebra to keep spine elastic and elongated; helps tone hips and legs; improves circulation; stimulates internal organs; eases problems of elimination and digestion.
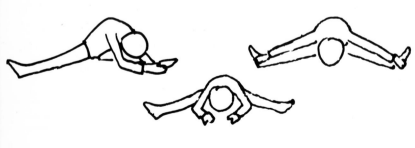 **LEG SPLITS**	Gives vigorous internal massage as body is pressed forward; stretches all muscles; increases elasticity of spine.

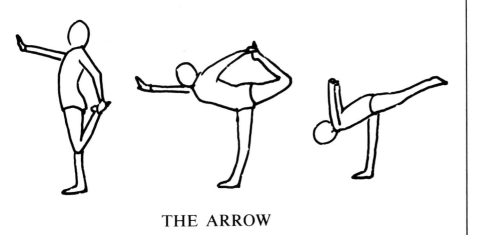

THE ARROW

Improves posture, balance and power of concentration; tones and firms entire body.

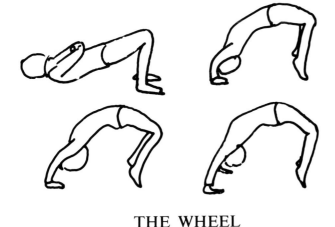

THE WHEEL

Develops strong back and arm muscles; when body is held high, arms, legs, spine and waist are toned and strengthened.

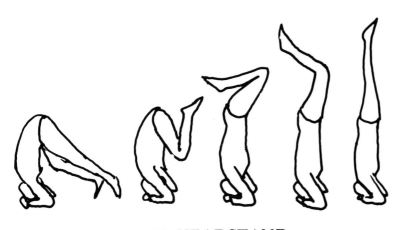

THE HEADSTAND

Puts body in perfect alignment; skin and facial tissues become nourished when a fresh supply of blood is sent to the head. Restores youth and vitality.

37. LOTUS POSTURE

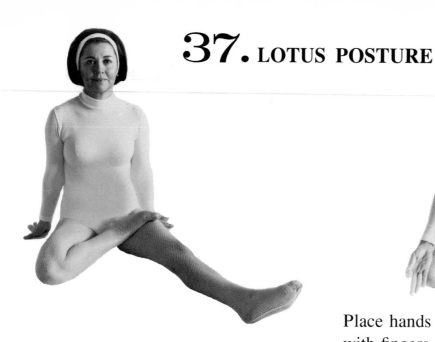
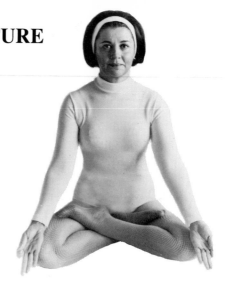

Sit with legs apart. Bend right knee and bring the foot over left thigh. Then bend left knee and bring foot over the right thigh. Don't be concerned if knees do not touch the floor. With practice they will limber.

Place hands over knees, palms up, with fingers in the "Symbol of Knowledge" pose. Hold for a few seconds while breathing deeply and calmly to distract your mind from the new stretch. Then bounce your legs up and down to stimulate circulation. Repeat, reversing the legs, with left over the right and right over the left.

---

38. BELLOWS BREATH

This exercise will take a little practice before you get the right rhythm. Emphasis is on forceful expulsion of the breath through the nose, similar to outward sniffs. Its staccato rhythm is deep, quick and vigorous.

Sit in one of the meditative postures with hands resting comfortably on the knees, or sit in a chair. Exhale forcefully through the nose, at the same time contracting abdomen to expel air with a powerful push from the diaphragm and thrust from the throat. Then release contraction and lungs will automatically take in air. Practice this exercise slowly to maintain an even rhythm, deep and forceful. Gradually build up to ten expulsions; then inhale deeply to fill the lungs with air, exhale and relax. This should take about 15 seconds. Repeat five times. When you are able to do ten expulsions with an even rhythm, then build up the expulsions to as many as possible.

39. THE PLOW AND VARIATIONS

For maximum benefit, hold each pose 5 seconds to increase the spine's elasticity and to tone the hips and legs.

Do not try to force your legs over the head so that toes will touch the floor. Do this slowly, and with practice the leg muscles will stretch sufficiently so that you can do the Plow and variations with more ease.

Lie flat on back with legs together, hands to sides, palms down, and eyes closed. Inhale; slowly raise legs over the head until toes touch the floor, or as far as they will reach. Exhale; breathe freely while holding the pose.

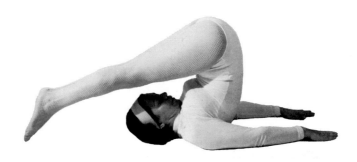

Spread legs apart and lock body with arms reaching over legs. Palms cover the ears. Hold the pose.

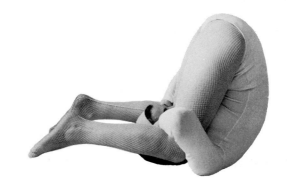

Raise arms over the head, straighten knees and draw legs together. Fingertips should touch toes. Hold. Without moving arms, use abdominal muscles to lower legs forward till they reach the floor. Then return arms to sides. Repeat three times.

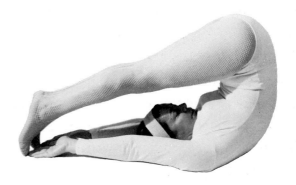

40. LEG SPLITS

These Leg Split variations will stretch most of the body muscles and give a vigorous internal massage as the body is pressed forward. Practice each step to gradually prepare yourself for more extensive limbering. Hold each pose for 5 seconds while breathing freely.

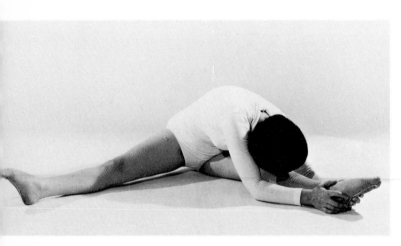

Sit with legs far apart. Inhale; bend forward to grasp left foot, elbows bent and head touching the knee, if possible. Hold to feel the stretch. Repeat same movements bending forward to grasp right foot.

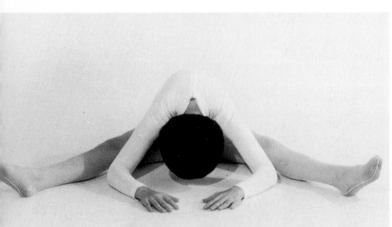

With legs far apart, inhale and bend forward, palms flat in front. Slide palms farther away from body as you lower your head to the floor. You should feel the pull in the spine and along inner thighs. Repeat three times.

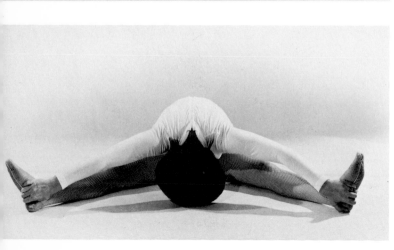

Then stretch arms out to grasp feet with head touching the floor. Repeat three times.

41. THE ARROW

The Arrow is a balance and concentration exercise, with two different poses. Each should be held for 15 to 20 seconds so that the entire body is stretched, toned and firmed, with the mind well focused on point of concentration.

Focus on an object within close distance. Stand on your right leg. Bend left leg behind and grasp it with your left hand. Inhale; raise right arm, stretching it out, palm up.

Exhale; slowly bend forward, moving left leg away from your body. Right arm and torso are on the same plane. Hold while breathing freely and concentrate on the arrow image. Repeat standing on your left leg.

While standing, interlock fingers behind back and slowly lower your body, at the same time raising left leg. Your body should slant downward with leg raised as high as possible to express the swiftness of the arrow on its journey. Hold while breathing freely, and concentrate on this thought. Repeat standing on your left leg.

42. THE WHEEL

The Wheel can be practiced either with feet flat on the floor or with heels raised. Since this exercise requires strong back and arm muscles to lift the torso, practice each step gradually to give your muscles time to strengthen. The Wheel is best done with bare feet to avoid sliding.

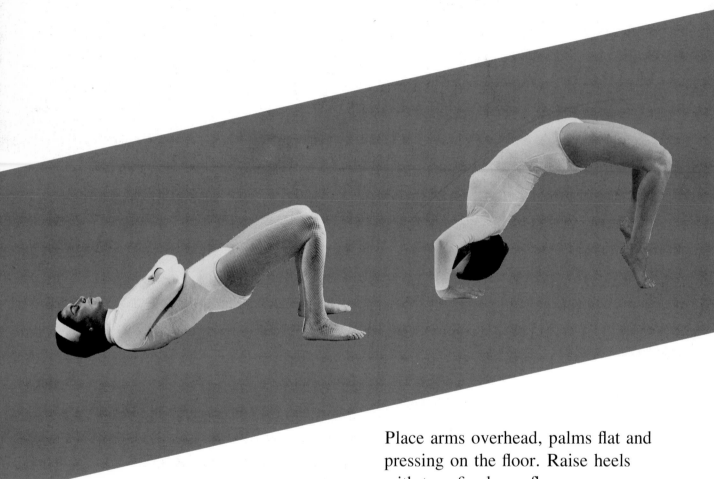

Lie on your back with knees bent, legs slightly apart, feet flat on the floor. Fold arms on chest. Inhale; raise buttocks off the floor as high as possible.

Place arms overhead, palms flat and pressing on the floor. Raise heels with toes firmly on floor, or keep heels flat.

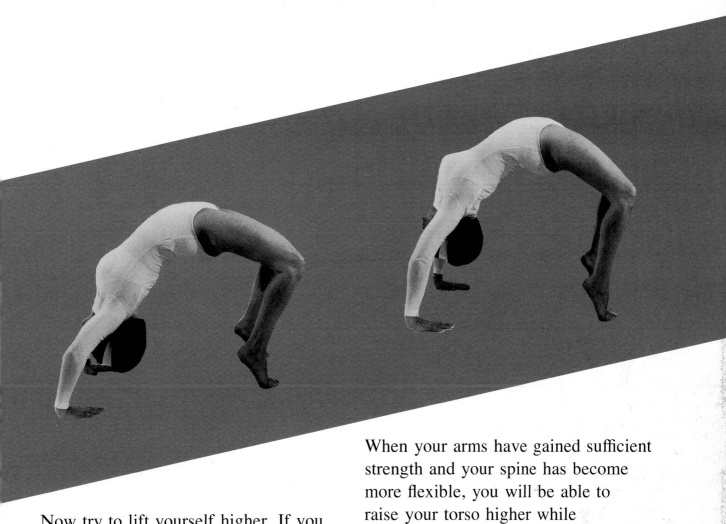

Now try to lift yourself higher. If you slide your head forward (away from your hands), you will be able to raise your torso in a bridge with palms and toes supporting your back.

When your arms have gained sufficient strength and your spine has become more flexible, you will be able to raise your torso higher while straightening arms to arch the spine, with head raised. Palms and toes (or feet) are firmly on the floor to avoid sliding. When you are in this position, hold for 10 to 15 seconds to feel the tremendous stretch in the spine, arms and legs. Repeat twice.

You may find you can do The Wheel without the first step, but this is a helpful way for anyone with weak back muscles. Both foot positions for The Wheel are shown in Exercise 51.

43. HEADSTAND

For self-confidence and safety, it is best to have someone nearby to help you in your first attempts with the Headstand. Use a wall as temporary support. When you gain control of your muscles and balance, you will no longer need support.

The Headstand should be practiced with caution. Before attempting to raise your legs in this inverted position, your neck and back muscles should be well strengthened by the preliminary steps given in Exercise 22. This will help you hold your body in correct position, and it will release any pressure at the base of the spine, in the sacral and lumbar regions. Your neck, too, will become limber and strong.

If you study the illustrations in Exercise 101, you will see how the body is supported while you are learning to raise your legs in the Headstand pose.

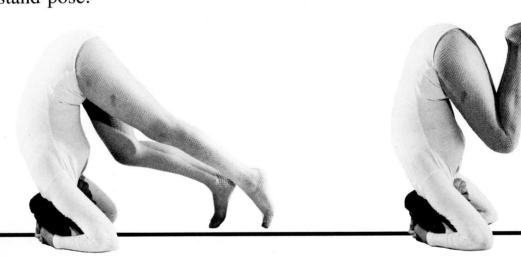

If you have been practicing the preliminary steps to the Headstand, your neck should be well strengthened. Continue to use a folded blanket or towel to support your head. Place it near a wall and continue to practice the "walk in" to the Headstand.

The next step is to bring your legs closer to your chest. Then bend your knees and try to raise your legs off the floor. This is a difficult step, and here is where you will need the assistance of someone to hold your back. Keep your knees close to your body with legs bent and toes pointing up. *Don't go any further until you are able to do this with sufficient control.* Once you have mastered this step, the rest will be easier.

Note: As long as your balance is unsteady, keep near a wall so you can reach for support. In this way you will not injure yourself. Also, learn to fall by relaxing all your muscles. If you find it easier at first to keep your eyes open to maintain your balance, then practice the Headstand this way. Eventually you will have no difficulty closing your eyes. When you are able to do the Headstand with control, repeat it three times and hold for a total of about 3 minutes. Don't be discouraged if it takes you several months before you make any noticeable progress in this posture. It is not an easy exercise, and some persons are able to balance more easily than others.

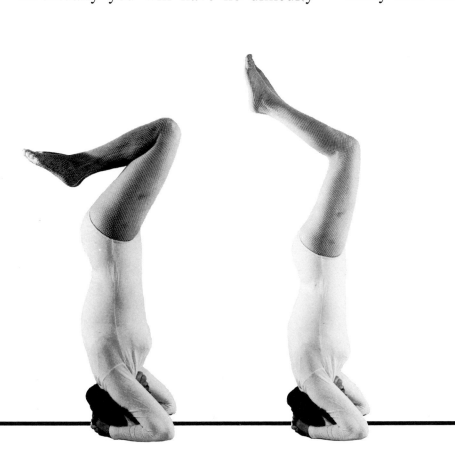

Then bend legs so that heels are above the buttocks. Be sure that your arms are firmly supporting your head with no strain on the neck. Your fingers should encircle the head and not be under it.

Raise legs a little higher with toes pointing upward. Keep arms firmly on the floor to support your head. Just before straightening the legs, tuck in the buttocks. Your spine should be straight to maintain perfect balance.

When your legs are vertical, toes pointing up, arms firmly supporting your head, you have achieved the Headstand. Have someone check your posture. When you come down from the Headstand reverse the steps, starting with Step 3. Remain in a lying position for a few seconds, then relax completely.

Congratulations! you have completed the Sixth Stage of this yoga course. Continue to practice those exercises which are still difficult for you to increase flexibility and keep your body slim and well toned. The combination of exercises suggested on page 153 will help vary your practice.

Chapter

3

VARIATIONS AND ADVANCED POSTURES

This chapter is actually an extension of A Yoga Course in Six Stages, since it consists mainly of variations of the basic postures, with a few new exercises.

As you delve deeper into yoga, you will discover that the variations are endless in challenging the human body to increase its flexibility and stamina. This is one good reason yoga has remained popular over a long period of time. It sustains interest and avoids monotony in physical exercises.

I have selected a group of teenagers to illustrate the postures in this chapter primarily to show what they are able to do after a brief introduction to yoga of a few weeks; some have had only a few hours of practice. They are not professional models—just young people who have found yoga an exciting way to keep physically fit.

44. THREE WAYS FOR THE ABDOMINAL LIFT

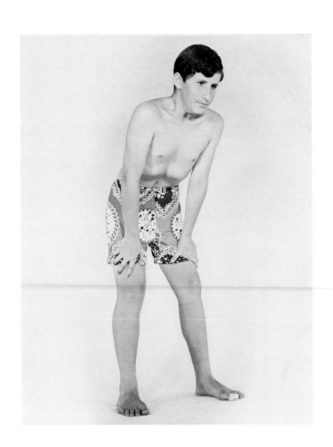

In all three poses the abdomen is pulled in and up toward back of the spine, and the diaphragm is drawn up, pressing against the rib cage. To create this vacuum, breathing is suspended after exhaling so that suction is possible. Refer to Exercise 9 for step-by-step instructions.

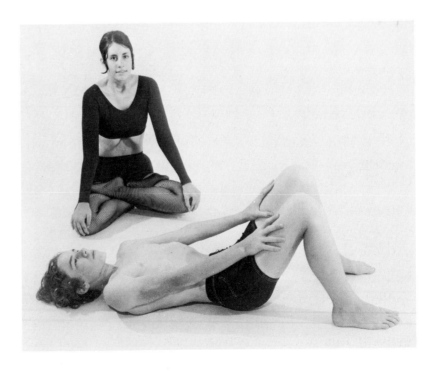

45. VARIATIONS OF THE CAMEL

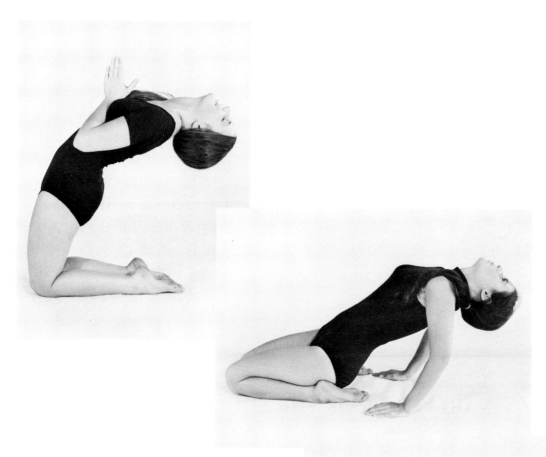

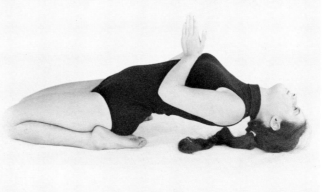

In the variation of The Camel in Step 1, palms are together over chest, and the pose is held for 5 seconds while breathing freely. See Exercise 11 for step-by-step instructions for the basic Camel. A more advanced pose of The Camel, in steps 2 and 3, will further develop flexibility of the spine, hips and knees. As thigh muscles are lengthened and toned, this will help to reduce hips and thighs. The second pose shows the necessary support, using palms placed down on floor, to lower head. There should be an arch between head and buttocks as in the third pose when body is in the supine position. Palms are together over the chest, and the pose is held for 5 seconds while breathing freely. To come up, place palms on floor for support.

46. VARIATION OF THE STOOP

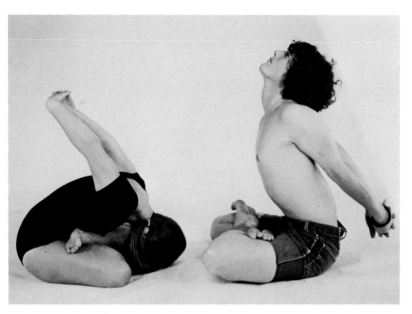

The traditional name for this posture is *Yoga Mudra*. It is done in the Lotus pose. The young man illustrates Step 1; and his companion completes the exercise in Step 2. Instructions for the breathing and bending movements are given in Exercise 24, a simple variation of this posture.

---

47. VARIATIONS OF THE SHOULDERSTAND

The Half-Lotus and Full Lotus in the Shoulderstand variations are a continuation of the series shown in Exercise 28.

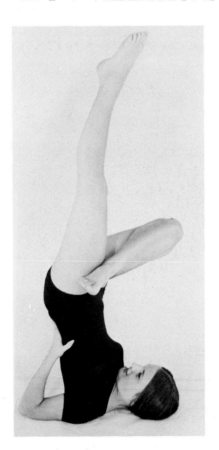

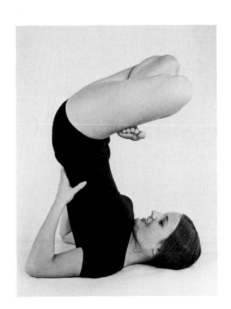

48. VARIATION OF THE INCLINED PLANE

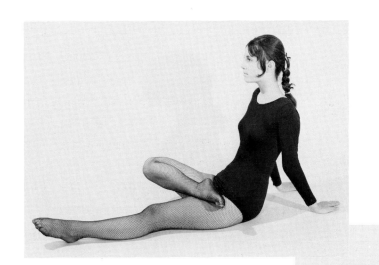

This is an advanced pose for the Inclined Plane given in Exercise 26. The only difference: right leg is bent over left thigh in a Half-Lotus pose. The rest of the exercise is the same as the simplified Inclined Plane.

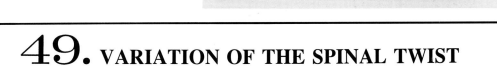

49. VARIATION OF THE SPINAL TWIST

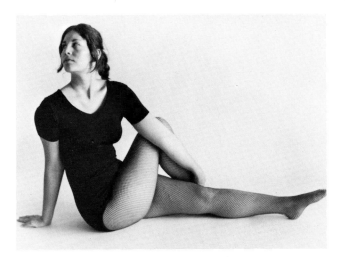

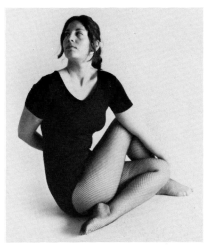

This advanced posture, known as the Full Spinal Twist, varies slightly from the simplified Half-Spinal Twist in Exercise 29. In this posture the left leg is bent back, with foot close to the right buttock. The rest of the exercise is the same as the simplified Spinal Twist.

50. VARIATION OF THE HALF-LOTUS POSTURE

In this variation of the basic Half-Lotus meditative pose, shown in Exercise 32, the right leg is bent back near the right buttock. The left foot is over the right thigh, close to the crotch. Arms are outstretched, with palms up, resting on the knees. Fingers form the "Symbol of Knowledge" pose. Repeat the same movements reversing the legs.
It is important to keep upper part of the body in perfect alignment. Spine, head and shoulders are held straight, ribs are lifted, and abdomen is held in. This pose will increase flexibility of the hips, knees and ankles, and is a preparatory exercise for the Lotus pose.

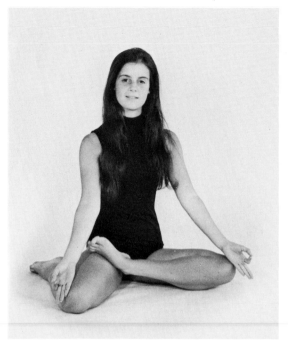

---

51. TWO VERSIONS OF THE WHEEL

At left, the body is raised in a high arch to form The Wheel while balanced on toes with palms firmly on the floor.

At right the traditional Wheel is shown with feet as well as palms flat on the floor. Complete instructions for this posture are given in Exercise 42.

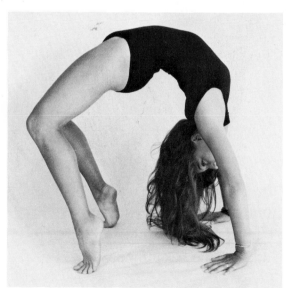

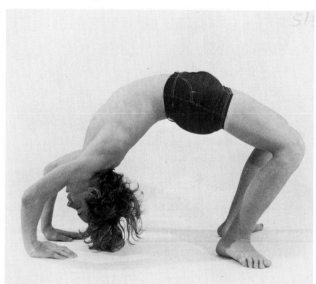

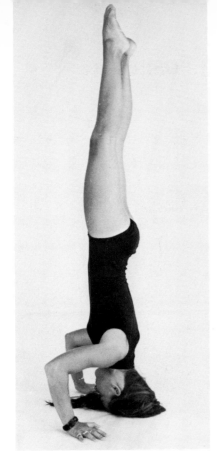

52. TRIPOD HEADSTAND

Some persons find the Tripod Headstand much easier to balance than the traditional way of clasping hands to encircle the head. Instructions for the Tripod Headstand are given in Exercise 102.

SEVEN NEW EXERCISES

53. SIDE BEND

This simple but effective exercise will slim the waistline and limber the legs. The left leg is bent, with foot close to the inner right thigh near the crotch. Right leg is bent back with foot close to the right buttock. Arms are over the head, with palms on top of each other. Spine is straight.

Inhale deeply while bending to the right. Hold about 3 seconds, exhale and bend over to the left. Hold again for 3 seconds. Repeat four times, alternating right and left. You should feel a pull in the waist.

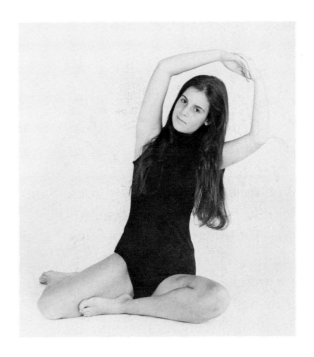

54. THE DANCER'S POSE

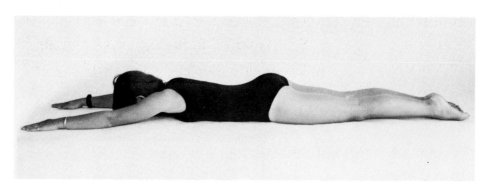

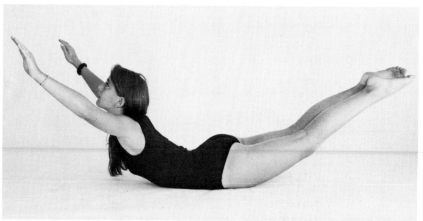

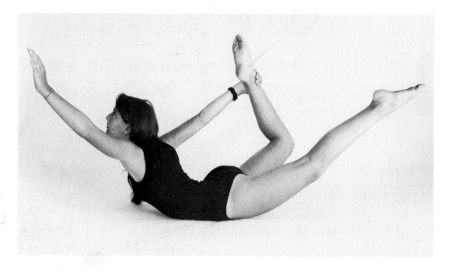

Well-toned arm and leg muscles and a flexible spine are needed to do this exercise properly.

Lie face down, arms and legs outstretched. Inhale and raise both arms and legs as high as possible. Breathing freely, grasp right ankle with right hand. Left arm and leg are still raised. Hold for 5 seconds, breathing freely, then relax and lower limbs. Repeat holding on to the left ankle with left hand. Do this exercise four times, alternating the right and left legs.

55. THE LOTUS FISH

Practice the Lotus posture with fingers forming the "Symbol of Knowledge" pose. Then place hands on floor as body bends back, head on floor with spine arched (see variation of the Lotus Fish in Exercise 96). Hold on to big toes with thumb and index fingers of both hands, which again form the "Symbol of Knowledge" pose. Repeat twice.

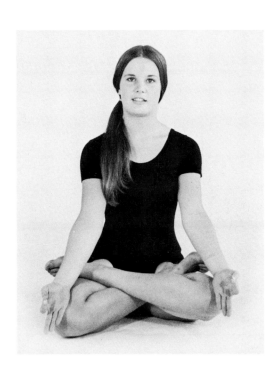

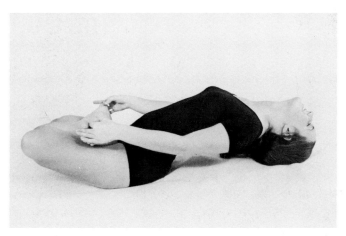

FOUR BALANCING EXERCISES

Practice of balancing postures given earlier in Exercises 14, 30 and 41 will be most helpful in carrying out these postures.

56. DEEP KNEE BEND

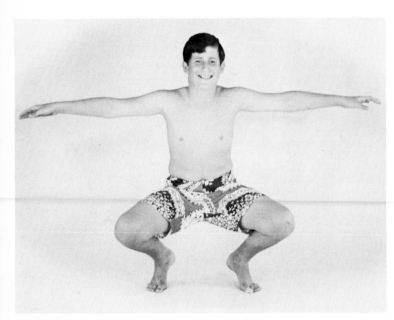

This exercise has a two-fold benefit: it develops balance and at the same time limbers and strengthens the knees and feet.

Stand with feet slightly apart and arms outstretched. Balance on toes. Inhale while lowering body, with spine straight, until knees are fully bent. Breathe freely and hold the pose for 5 seconds. Repeat three times.

58. THE EAGLE

The balancing Eagle is an excellent exercise to tone and limber muscles of the legs and arms. Stand on left leg. Twist right leg around it. Entwine arms in front of chest, right elbow tucked in the left with palms over each other; fingers touch nose. When balance is secure, inhale and bend forward until elbows rest on right thigh or knee. Keep arms entwined with fingers touching nose. Hold for 5 seconds, breathing freely. Relax. Repeat same movements standing on right leg and twisting the left around it. Do this exercise four times, alternating the right and left legs.

▶

57. ONE-LEG STAND

In this balancing posture, the head, body and left leg are on an even plane, with the right leg firmly supporting the weight. To practice this exercise, stand with feet together, arms clasped behind head, spine straight. Inhale while slowly bending forward, at the same time raising the left leg until you are on an even plane. Breathe freely and hold the pose for 5 seconds. Relax and repeat standing on the left leg. Do this exercise four times, alternating the left and right legs.

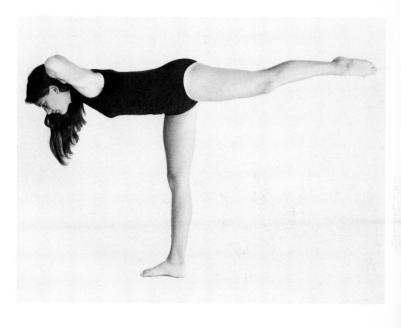

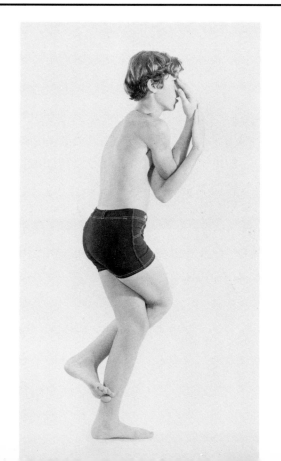

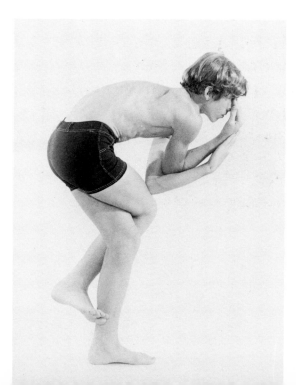

59. THE CROW

The balancing Crow requires strength in the arms and wrists to support weight of the body when legs are raised. Since this exercise takes a great deal of practice before balance is secure to raise the legs, as a protection place a pillow on the floor between hands, just in case you fall.

First squat on toes, legs apart, with palms flat on floor. Elbows are slightly bent and close to inner part of knees. Inhale; press elbows against knees, then try to raise your legs. Breathe freely while holding the pose for 5 seconds, or as long as possible. Repeat three times.

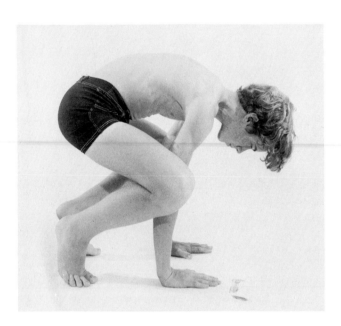

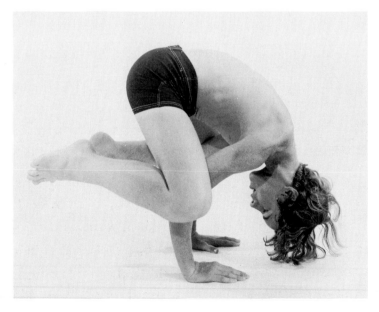

Chapter

4

EXERCISES YOU CAN DO IN A CHAIR

These exercises, designed to be done in a chair, tone and limber all parts of the body, from head to toe. Their advantage is that almost anyone can do them, anywhere, anytime: at the office, at home, traveling or vacationing. The elderly and those physically restricted will find these exercises a painless way to firm up flabby muscles and redistribute body weight.

The only requirements are to loosen any clothing that is tight around the waist, to keep the spine straight (or as straight as possible), and to remove your shoes. Rest your feet a few inches apart, flat on the floor.

60. HEAD ROLL

When tension builds up in the back of the neck, the Head Roll will loosen tight muscles.

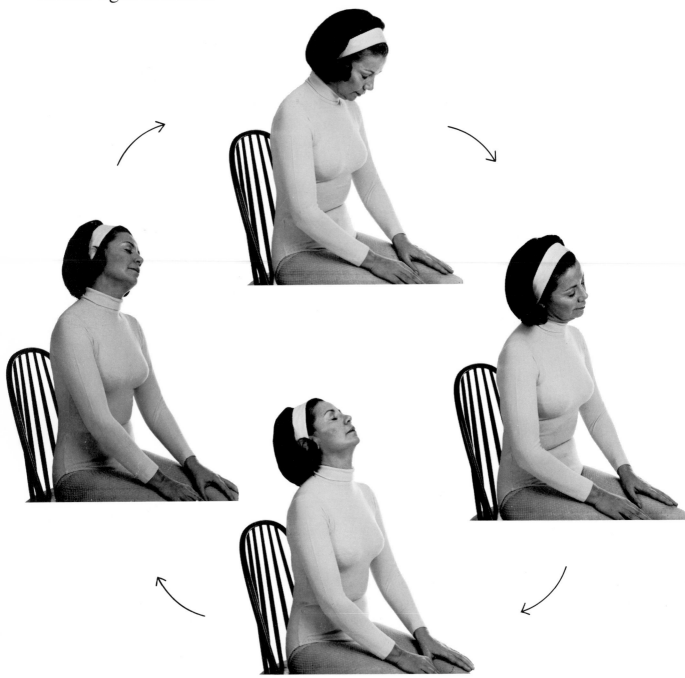

Roll your head loosely in a circle: forward and down, right, back, left and forward again. Repeat three times slowly without stopping, then reverse the motion: forward and down, left, back, right and forward again. Repeat three times slowly without stopping. Relax.

61. FOR TENSE SHOULDERS AND TO ACHIEVE BETTER POSTURE

These simple rotating movements will relieve tense muscles in the back, neck and shoulders.

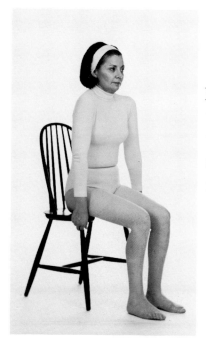

Bring shoulders forward, raise them up, arch them back, and then lower. Repeat five times slowly, holding each movement about 5 seconds.

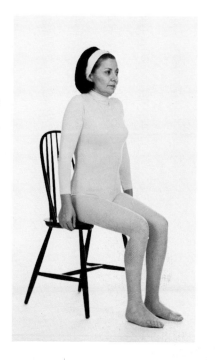

If you have a tendency to slouch, do this exercise:

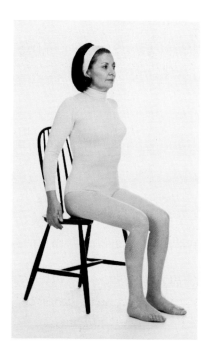

Arch shoulders back to contract back muscles as at left. Hold for 20–30 seconds to feel cross pull in the back. Relax and repeat five times.

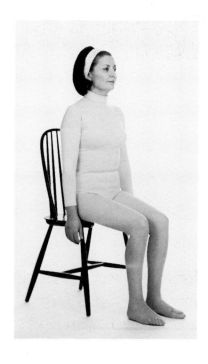

62. FOR PAINFUL FINGER JOINTS AND WRISTS

Do these exercises as often as necessary to relax stiff joints.

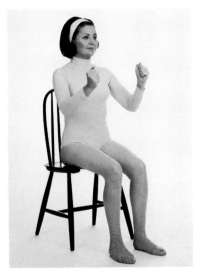

For finger joints, make fists
with both hands, elbows
bent.
Forcefully fling fingers apart.

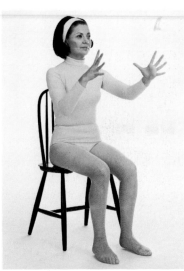

Then slowly draw them
inward, using resistance,
until you form fists again.

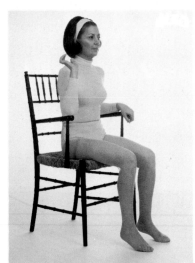

For the wrist, rest elbow on
arm of chair. With hand
relaxed, rotate wrist in a
circle five times to the right,
five times to the left. Repeat
separately with each wrist.

63. BACK STRETCH

If you have a tendency to slouch, the Back Stretch will improve your posture. It is also a limbering exercise for arms and shoulders.

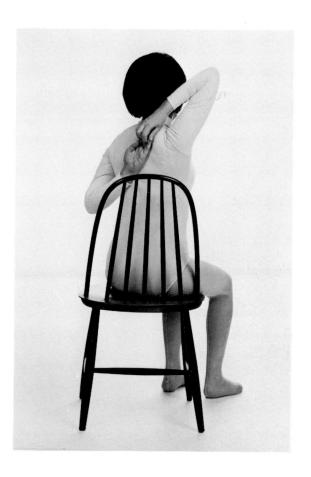

Raise right arm and bend it back over right shoulder with palm flat, just below the neck. Cross left hand behind the back, with back of hand resting on the spine, fingers upward. Now try to make the fingertips meet. With practice, as the muscles are stretched, you will be able to lock your fingers.

Keep your arms in this position, head straight. Inhale deeply (expanding your abdomen) and contract back muscles to feel the pull. Keep stretching to bring both hands closer together, but don't strain. Exhale, arms down, and relax.

Repeat four times, alternating right and left arms over the shoulder, with the other behind the back.

64. FOR WEAK BACK MUSCLES

The play of resistance in this exercise has many benefits. It reduces the buttocks, firms arms and strengthens weak back muscles.

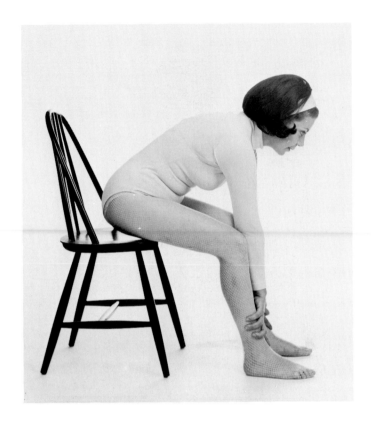

Lean forward to grasp your legs as far down as possible. Then, with the breath held and still grasping the legs, pull straight up, using only back muscles. You should feel the pull in your buttocks, arms and back. Hold for 5–10 seconds. Repeat three times.

65. ABDOMINAL LIFT

One of the best ways to stimulate intestinal activity and strengthen muscles of the abdomen is by doing the abdominal lift. This exercise should be done at least two hours after you have eaten. Remove or loosen any clothing that binds the waist.

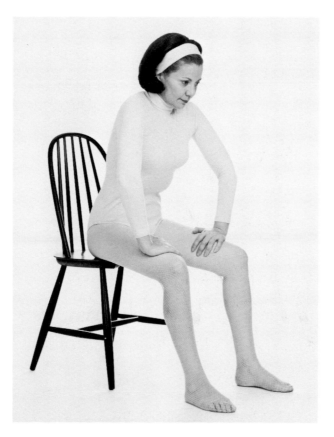

Sit with spine straight, body leaning slightly forward, legs apart, hands pressing on your inner thighs. Inhale deeply through the nose, then vigorously exhale through the mouth in a "ha" sound. This will empty the lungs and create a vacuum in the abdominal cavity. Hold your breath and draw up the diaphragm, pressing it against the rib cage, so that the abdomen is pulled in and up toward the spine. Hold for 10–20 seconds without breathing. Relax. Repeat three times.

When the abdominal muscles have been strengthened through the lift, practice the pumping movement by pulling in the abdominal muscles, then forcefully thrusting them out, five to ten times while holding the breath. Repeat three times.

For three views of the Abdominal Lift in action, see Exercise 44.

66. TONING ARMS, CHEST AND SHOULDERS

The Horizontal and Vertical Stretches stimulate circulation through deep breathing, and the play of resistance tones muscles in the upper arms, chest and shoulders. Each exercise is repeated three times *while holding your breath for approximately twenty seconds.* Sit with feet slightly apart and spine straight.

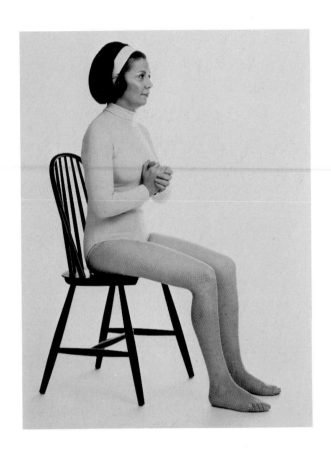
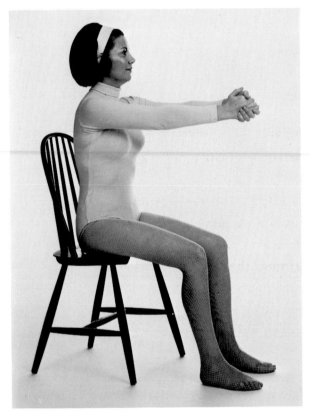

Horizontal Stretch

Clasp hands close to chest. Inhale deeply (expanding abdomen). Then stretch arms forward. While holding your breath, use resistance to slowly pull arms toward you, touching the chest. Repeat three times, then exhale and relax.

Vertical Stretch

Clasp hands behind head. Inhale deeply (expanding abdomen). Then stretch arms upward. While holding your breath, use resistance to slowly pull arms down behind the head, touching back of neck. Repeat three times, then exhale and relax.

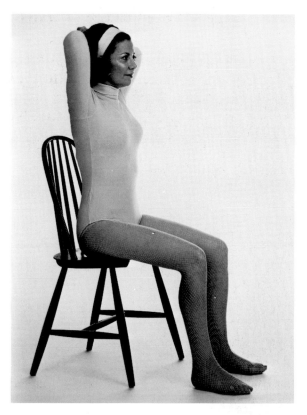

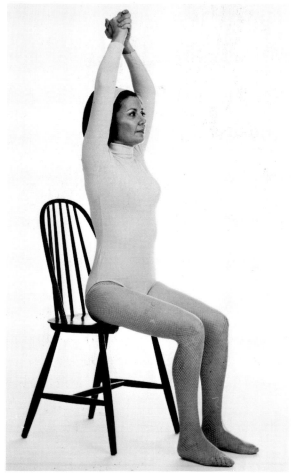

67. BEAUTY TREATMENT FOR THE FACE (The Lion Pose)

Practice this invigorating facial exercise before a mirror to see the effect of muscles in action. Called in yoga the Lion pose, facial movements imitate the fierceness of a lion springing; this prevents the sagging of facial and neck muscles. Emphasis is on the forceful expulsion of breath through the mouth; then the breath is held for a few seconds as the muscles are pulled taut.

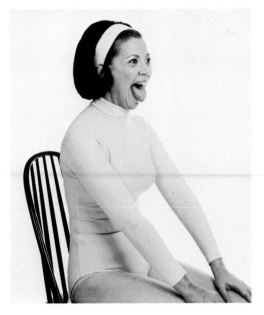

Inhale deeply; then forcefully exhale through your mouth. While exhaling with mouth wide open and eyes wide and staring, thrust out your tongue and stretch arms down with fingers stiff and spread tautly apart. Hold the breath for a few seconds. Then close your mouth and inhale deeply through the nostrils (expanding the abdomen). Exhale again slowly through your nostrils and relax. Repeat three times.

---

68. TONING NECK AND CHIN LINE

These movements, done slowly with deliberate force, limber tight muscles at back of neck, and also tone throat and chin line.

Place clasped hands on your forehead, elbows out. Press backward, using resistance. Repeat three times.

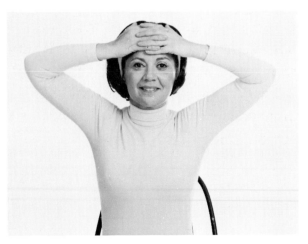

69. FIRMING BUSTLINE AND STRENGTHENING CHEST

Through play of resistance in these movements, you should feel the pull in the arms, chest and shoulders.

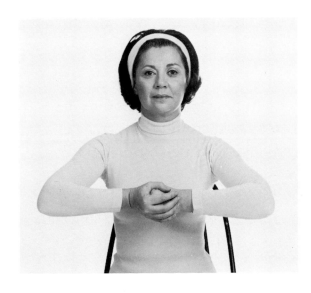

Sit straight with arms held across the chest. Place one fist inside the palm of the other hand. Press hands together, using forcible strength of arms and shoulders.
Repeat three times.

70. FIRMING UNDERSIDES OF ARMS

Flabby undersides of the arms will quietly firm if you do this exercise faithfully. You should feel the pull in the shoulders and lower surface of the arms.

Sit straight with feet flat on the floor. Grasp the bottom edge of the chair with fingertips of both hands. Then try to lift the chair, exerting as much strength as possible, while holding your breath and using resistance. Repeat three times.

71. FIRMING LEGS, ABDOMEN AND BUTTOCKS

Play of resistance is the key to this exercise.

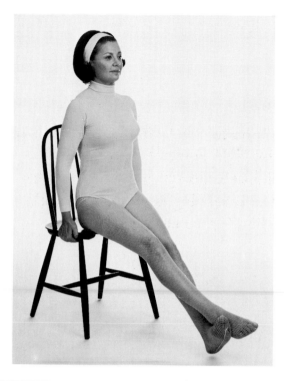

Sit with legs rigidly outstretched and crossed at the ankles. Hold on to the seat of your chair and try to pull your feet apart, using resistance. Repeat three times.

---

72. FIRMING INNER THIGHS

Hard-to-firm inner thigh muscles will respond to this exercise.

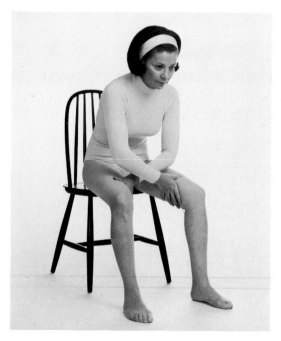

Lean slightly forward in a chair with feet a few inches apart. Cross arms and place hands inside opposite knees. Then try to press knees together, using resistance. Hold for 5–10 seconds. Repeat three times.

73. FOR WEAK KNEES

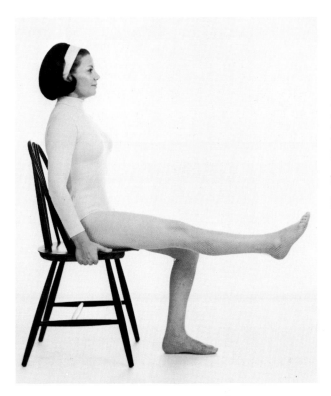

Hold on to chair with feet flat on floor. Raise right leg till knee is straight. Contract kneecap by pulling muscles upward, keeping knee straight. Hold for 15–20 seconds.

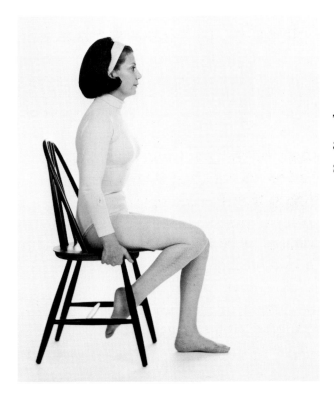

Then bend leg down under chair as far as you can. Repeat five times. Repeat same movements with left leg.

74. SLIMMING ANKLES AND STRENGTHENING ARCHES

These exercises should be done with shoes off.

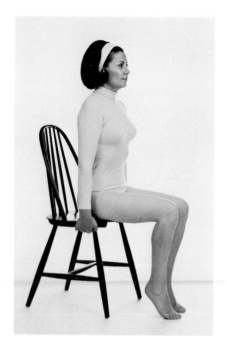

To slim ankles, hold on to sides of chair. Raise heels, toes resting on the floor. Press down on toes. The higher you raise heels with toes on floor, the more pull you will feel in the insteps and ankles. Repeat five times. Hold for 15–20 seconds, using resistance.

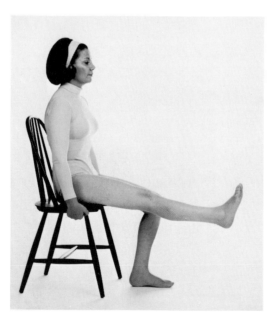 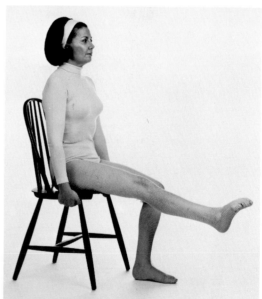

To strengthen arches of feet and relieve tired muscles, raise foot about 10 inches off the floor. Curl toes under foot. Hold for 15–20 seconds. Repeat five times. Lower leg and repeat with left foot.

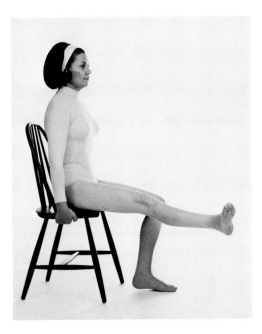

To strengthen ankles, raise right foot about 10 inches off the floor. Rotate it slowly with ankle relaxed: five times to the right, five times to the left. Lower leg. Repeat with left foot.

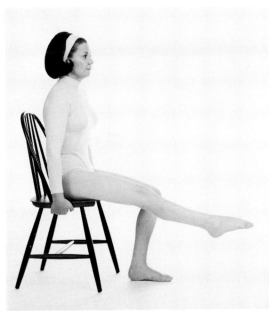

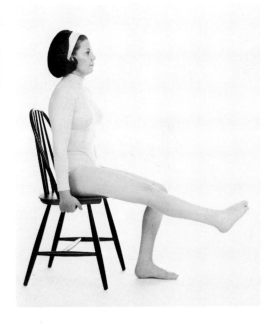

75. PALMING

Palming is one of the best ways to relax the sensory nerves and reduce eyestrain. It helps you see better for longer periods of time and also has calming effect on the mind. The more relaxed you are when your eyes are closed, the darker will be the field of vision. Remove eyeglasses when doing this exercise.

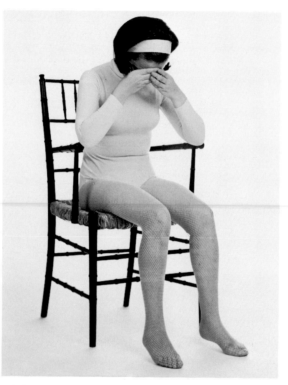

Sit in a comfortable position where your elbows can rest on the arms of a chair or on a table. Briskly rub the heels of your palms to charge them with electricity. Then cover eyes with cupped hands. Heels of palms rest on the cheekbones with fingers crossed over the forehead. Palms should not touch eyeballs. Close your eyes without pressing the eyelids. At first you will see bright spots, then gray. The more relaxed you are, the darker will be your vision.

To completely relax, create a mental image of a particularly restful place you have visited. You can think of a brook and the trickling of water on the smooth pebbles. Direct your mind to this peaceful scene, and dismiss all extraneous thoughts. Think only of the brook and how delightfully calm and tranquil it is. The deeper your concentration, the better you are able to hold this image and the more relaxed you will become. Your field of vision is growing darker and darker. Now take a deep breath, open your eyes and look around you. Everything you see will appear sharper and clearer. This flash of improved vision will come more frequently with the practice of palming.

Chapter

5

YOGA FOR CHILDREN

Yoga is a natural form of exercise for children. Their supple bodies respond to poses with which they can identify, such as the postures imitating animals, insects, birds and fish. With little or no effort, most children can uncoil like a cobra or become a swan, an eagle, a grasshopper, a tree, an archer or a mountain. And without their realizing it, through these exercises they will further limber their joints and develop muscle control, coordination, physical poise and concentration.

But not all children are fortunate enough to be born limber with good coordination. A little girl of five—to the surprise of her mother, who is a ballet dancer—could not bend her knees without feeling a twinge of pain; a boy of six showed signs of a rigid spine, and another boy of nine was faced with two problems: overweight and lack of coordination. For such a child the cardinal rule is *never to push him beyond his abilities.* Let the coaxing be gentle and the atmosphere cheerful. Usually the child responds and enjoys the game-like sessions, and he is often helped immeasurably.

While a child's body is still limber, or can be made so with little effort, is the time to introduce a series of yoga exercises he will enjoy and which can become part of a daily routine.

The benefits of yoga have been recognized by many elementary schools in Europe, and yoga exercises with deep breathing have become part of their physical-culture curriculum. Hopefully, more schools in the United States will realize what yoga can do for children and will incorporate it into their programs for physical health.

According to Dr. Philip Rice in his book *Building for Mental and Physical Health*, "The I.Q. of a child can be increased by enlarging his intake of oxygen through correct deep breathing." Unfortunately, this is not the way children are taught to breathe in gym classes. "Take a deep breath—stomach in! chest out!" is the usual instruction—which leads to upper-chest breathing and is the reverse of diaphragmatic breathing.

Parents might think about starting a small yoga group of their child's friends. The successive exercises given in this chapter will serve as the basis of a teaching program. Parents or teachers who have followed A Yoga Course in Six Stages in Chapter 2, will have acquired sufficient knowledge to teach the postures and correct breathing to children.

Yoga should be taught in gradual stages, without forcing the child to stretch or bend beyond his limitation. Ten minutes is about the maximum for a yoga session to sustain the interest of a child as young as five. Those older than seven are able to take about 15 minutes. But children will rapidly lose interest the moment they feel they are being pushed beyond their endurance or if the lessons are dull.

Working with children is a gratifying experience. Results are often immediate. In a short time they are able to do complicated postures, such as The Tortoise, The Diving Swan, The Lotus Fish and The Archer, which require ultimate flexibility. Adults achieve these postures only after years of practice. With their imaginative love of make-believe, children enjoy yoga and respond in astonishing ways to the characteristics of each posture. The wonderful thing about yoga is that the postures lend themselves to characters from well-known fables, such as "The Hare and the Tortoise" (see Exercises 80 and 97). This opens up a creative approach to teaching the postures, and the combinations are endless.

If you wish to increase the range of exercises for children, add some of the postures from Chapter 2. But it is important to realize that while children generally are extremely limber and can do some of the most complicated physical postures, such as The Tortoise or The Lotus Fish, they do not have the muscle control of teen-agers or adults. For instance, they should not be taught breathing techniques beyond those given in this chapter that require more control of the diaphragm, nor should they be given difficult balancing exercises or any postures that call for muscle control beyond a child's ability.

Children, like adults, can vary in their suppleness, and the parent should recognize what each child is able to do and gently help him in those exercises he finds difficult. Whatever a child's physical ability, yoga will develop better coordination and poise, and it is one way all children can remain healthy and limber for the rest of their lives if they spend just ten minutes a day in the practice of yoga.

The children whose pictures appear in this book have had not more than 5 hours of yoga. They are not professional models—simply children who were given the opportunity to be introduced to yoga.

76. THE BALLOON
First Step in Deep Breathing

When guiding children to the first step in diaphragmatic breathing, let them imagine that breathing is like blowing a balloon. When they breathe in, air fills the tummy, which is blown out like a balloon. When they breathe out and no air is left in the tummy, it becomes as flat as a balloon without any air.

The boy in the background is inhaling as his tummy is "blown out"; his companion is exhaling as he pulls his tummy in, making it flat.

This breathing exercise should be done five times slowly without stopping so that the child can feel a sense of rhythm.

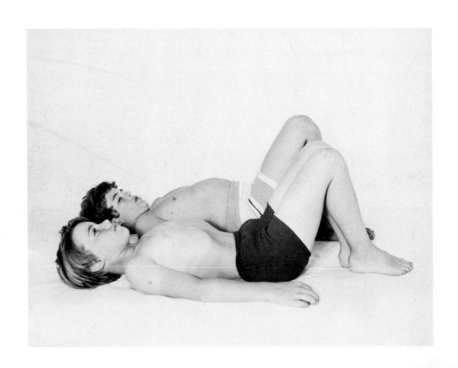

77. THE ROOSTER
Second Step in Deep Breathing

The second step in deep breathing has been turned into an imitation of a balancing-crowing rooster. Children love to utter the call of a rooster while they flutter their imaginary wings and, at the same time, hold their balance on tiptoe.

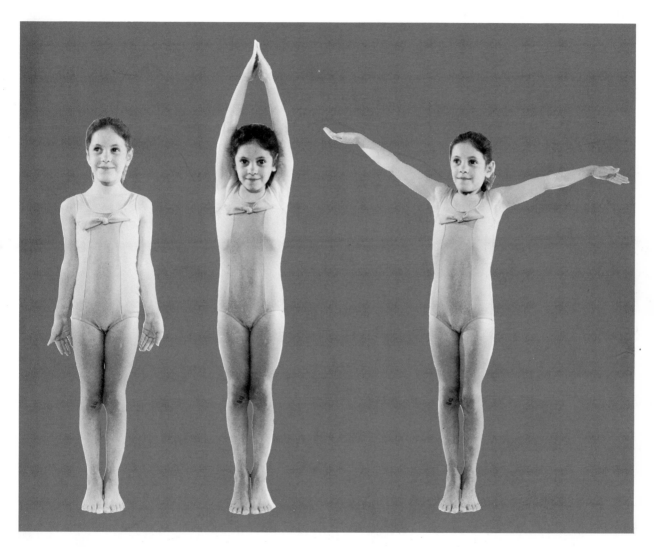

Stand with feet together, spine straight, arms down with palms turned out.

Inhale deeply (blowing tummy out) while raising arms overhead, palms touching. Exhale (tummy pulled in) while slowly dropping arms to sides.

Inhale, balance on toes, and spread arms out at sides. Then breathe freely and balance for a few seconds, at the same time fluttering arms as if they were wings. Repeat three times.

78. THREE LITTLE FROGS

These different poses of The Frog are primarily for balance, good posture, and limbering of the legs. Some children are unable to lower their knees to the floor as in the Sitting Frog pose. *Do not push.* You will find the stretching practice given in the next exercise helpful for gradual limbering.

Repeat each exercise three times.

The Squatting Frog

Squat with legs spread far apart so that toes are close to buttocks. Keep spine straight. Hands are placed on knees.

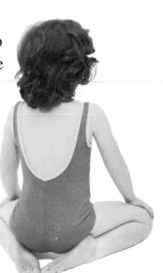

The Balancing Frog

Balance with weight of body resting on heels, spine straight. When balance is steady, fold arms overhead.

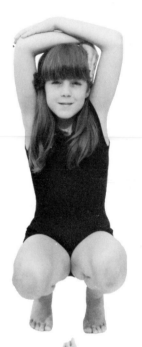

The Sitting Frog

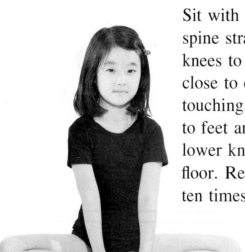

Sit with legs apart, spine straight. Bend knees to bring feet close to crotch, soles touching. Hold on to feet and try to lower knees to the floor. Repeat ten times.

Sit with legs spread far apart with soles of feet touching close to crotch, knees resting on the floor. Raise hands and join palms overhead, fingertips touching.

79. THE FLOATING FISH

The Fish is a favorite exercise of anyone who tries it. Children love it because they can imagine that they are little fish floating in a cool mountain stream. Adults find it a relaxing exercise while it strengthens the back and neck muscles. In addition, when the back is arched, the chest is thrown open for deeper and fuller breathing. The traditional name of this posture is The Half-Fish. It is a simplified version of The Lotus Fish in Exercise 96.

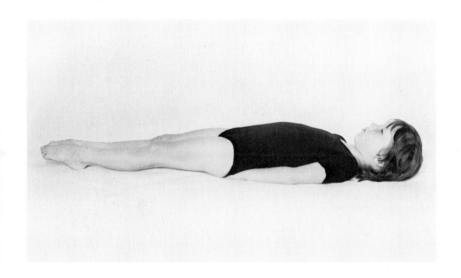

Lie flat on back with legs together, palms down under buttocks, eyes closed. Inhale; raise chest off the floor, using elbows for support, to create a bridge between the top of head and lower back. While breathing freely, hold the pose a few seconds. Then lower head and chest and slowly return to the first position. Repeat three times.

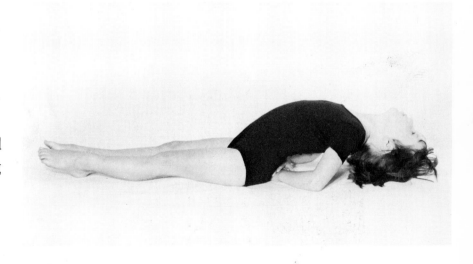

80. THE HARE

Simple as this posture may appear, its benefits are many. When the head is lowered to the floor (with chin touching the jugular notch), and the pose held for a few seconds, a fresh supply of blood is sent to the brain. Also, when the body is in this pose, the spine is stretched and limbered. Hands remain grasping the feet throughout the exercise. This is a good exercise for both children and adults.

Sit on heels with legs together, spine straight. Hold feet with hands.

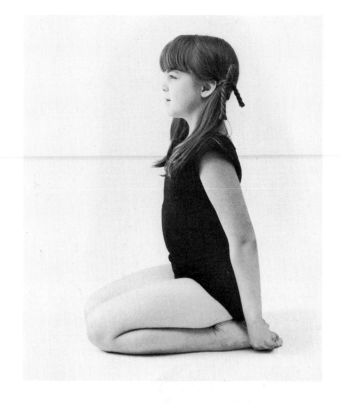

Inhale and slowly bend forward until head is lowered to the floor near knees. Chin should touch jugular notch, or close to it. Arms are still stretched to grasp the feet. Exhale, breathe freely, and hold the pose a few seconds, then return to the Kneeling Hare position. Repeat three times.

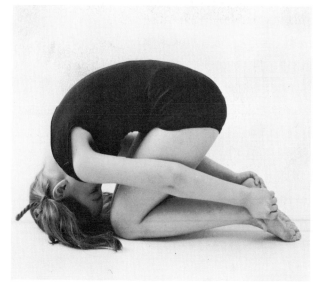

81. THE WOODCHOPPER

This vigorous movement of a woodchopper swinging down to strike with an imaginary ax is a favorite with children—especially boys, for whom the bracing action releases pent-up energy. Adults will find this exercise a good way to limber the spine.

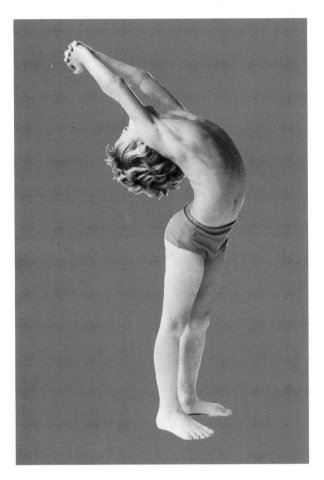

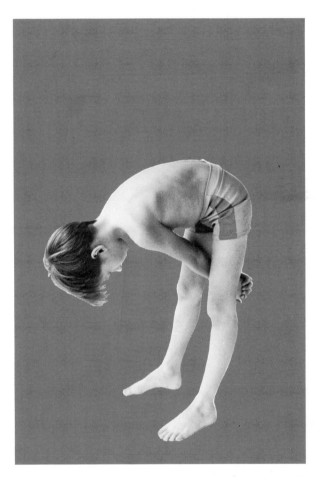

Swinging Back. Stand with feet wide apart, hands clasped in front with fingers interlocked. Inhale, raise arms up and overhead, bend back until spine and neck are arched.

Swinging Down. Exhale. With a vigorous swing come forward and down, hands between legs, as if you were actually chopping wood. Breathe freely and let arms swing back and forth between legs five or six times before raising them up overhead again. Repeat three times.

82. THE COBRA

The slow uncoiling movements of The Cobra will develop strong back muscles as the spine rolls back, vertebra by vertebra. Adults should do this exercise with elbows bent for additional toning of the spine. Hips rest on the floor.

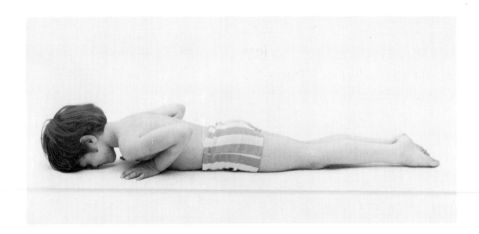

The Sleeping Cobra. Lie face down with forehead touching the floor, arms bent with palms close to chest, legs together.

The Striking Cobra. Inhale and slowly raise torso, keeping hips on floor. When arms are almost stretched, arch neck back. Exhale. While breathing freely, hold the pose a few seconds to feel the stretch in the spine. Then slowly lower chest and arms until head touches the floor. Repeat twice.

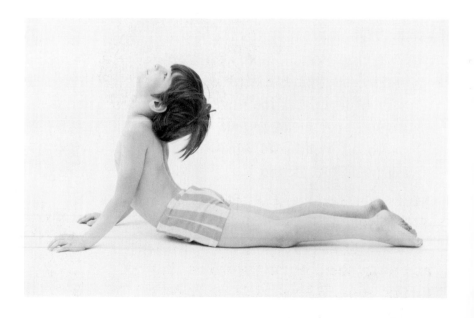

83. THE CAT

This delightful sequence of stretching the entire body resembles the graceful movements of a cat. Children put it at the top of their list of favorites. Adults will find the sequence of stretches a pleasant way to limber the body and develop poise. For maximum stretch, hands should remain in the same position throughout the sequence. Hold each pose a few seconds while breathing freely.

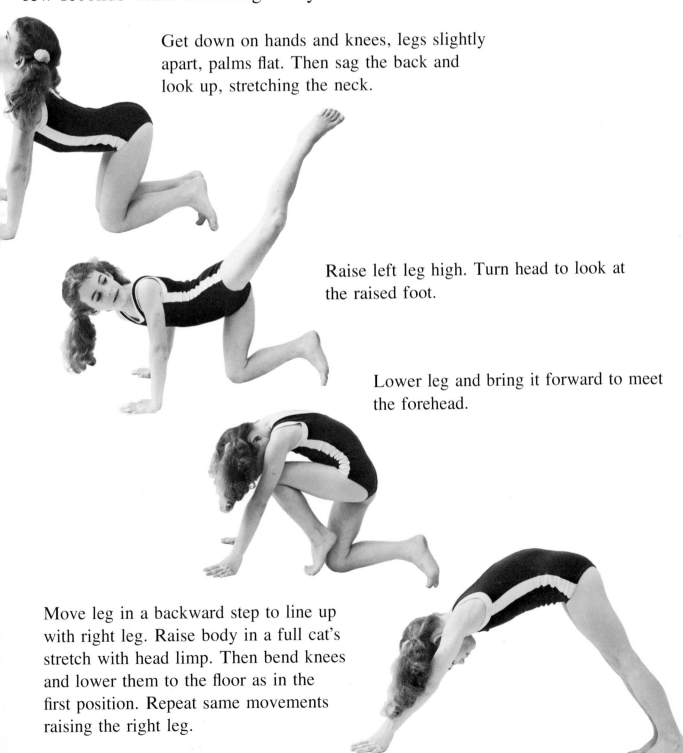

Get down on hands and knees, legs slightly apart, palms flat. Then sag the back and look up, stretching the neck.

Raise left leg high. Turn head to look at the raised foot.

Lower leg and bring it forward to meet the forehead.

Move leg in a backward step to line up with right leg. Raise body in a full cat's stretch with head limp. Then bend knees and lower them to the floor as in the first position. Repeat same movements raising the right leg.

84. THE SWAN

These graceful swanlike movements are a stretching exercise to keep the spine limber and improve the posture. The key to The Swan is to keep the palms flat on the floor as the body moves from the Rising to the Resting Swan pose. This is a beneficial exercise for all ages.

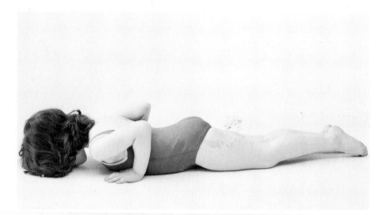

The Sleeping Swan. Lie face down with forehead touching the floor, elbows bent and palms flat just below chest level.

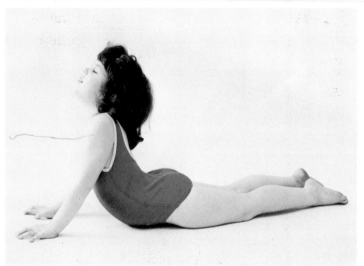

The Rising Swan. Inhale; slowly raise head and chest until arms are fully stretched with head bent back.

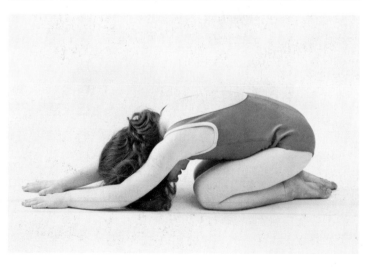

The Resting Swan. Exhale; without lifting palms from floor, slowly sit back on heels, arms outstretched in front and forehead touching the floor. Breathe freely and hold the pose a few seconds to feel the stretch. Then, without lifting the palms, move up and forward, returning to the Rising Swan pose. Slowly lower chest and arms until head touches the floor as in the first pose. Repeat twice.

85. THE CAMEL

This sequence of camel-like movements will keep the spine, hips, knees and ankles limber. Children generally have no difficulty doing them. Some adults, however, find the movements too challenging if the spine and knee joints are stiff. In that case each movement should be practiced gradually to induce further limbering of the body. (See Exercise 11.)

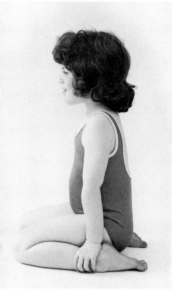

The Sitting Camel. Sit on floor with legs slightly apart and buttocks resting on heels. Grasp ankles to support back, spine straight.

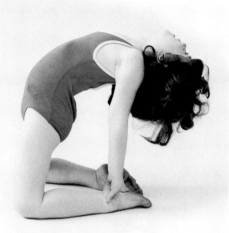

The Kneeling Camel. Raise body to arch spine in a kneeling position. Bend back until hands grasp ankles with neck arched back and relaxed.

The Resting Camel. Return to the Sitting Camel pose, then bend back until head touches the floor with buttocks resting on heels. Place hands on thighs. Spine is arched to create a bridge between head and buttocks.

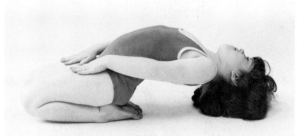

The Sleeping Camel. Return to the Sitting Camel pose (press palms on floor to give you a lift). Bend forward, head touching floor, with buttocks resting on heels and hands grasping feet. Then sit up as in the first position. Repeat twice.

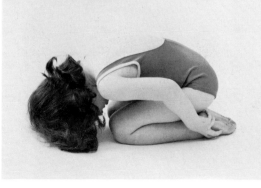

86. THE SWALLOW

These imaginary poses of a swallow taking flight are actually deep-breathing and stretching exercises.

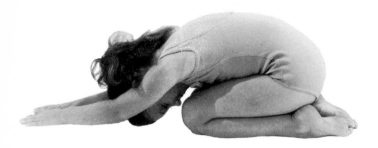

Sit on heels with head bent forward to the floor, arms outstretched and resting limply in front of the head with palms flat.

Inhale; slowly rise up to a kneeling position, bend back, and stretch arms overhead.

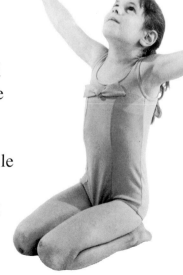

Exhale; bend forward, tipping head down. Bring arms up and out at the sides and imagine them to be the wings of a swallow taking flight. Breathe freely. Let arms flutter while pose is held a few seconds. Then slowly return to the original resting pose. Repeat twice.

87. THE STORK

This is a simple lesson in balance and concentration.

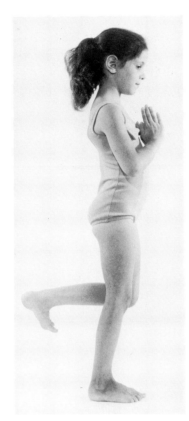

Stand on right foot with left knee bent so that foot is at knee level from the floor. Bend elbows, with palms touching close to chest (left). Then bring head down to meet palms, symbolizing a sleeping stork (right). Balance for a few seconds, keeping perfectly still. Repeat standing on left foot with right knee bent back. When balance is secure, this posture should be done with eyes closed and the balance held for a few seconds.

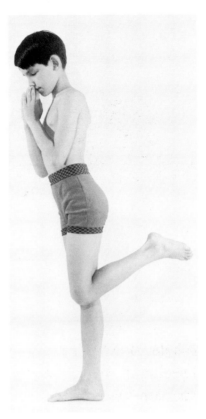

88. BIRD IN FLIGHT

This imaginary posture of a bird in flight develops poise, balance and concentration. Breathing is free. Eyes are open.

Balance on toes. Bend forward with arms straight back, body perfectly poised. Hold a few seconds, keeping as still as possible. Repeat three times.

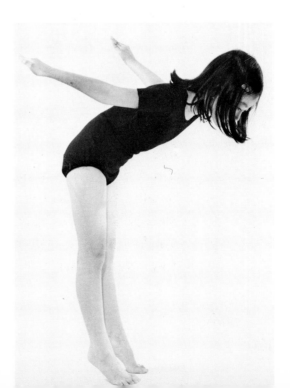

89. THE SHOULDERSTAND AND PLOW IN ONE

Most children are able to do these postures with little practice. When their back muscles become strengthened in the Shoulderstand pose, they will be able to hold their legs up with knees straight; the stretch of the hamstring muscles in the Plow pose will enable them eventually to keep their legs straight and toes on the floor. See Exercise 21 for step-by-step explanation of the Shoulderstand.

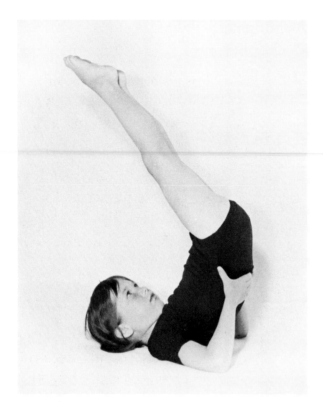

In the Shoulderstand pose, legs are raised over the head with knees straight. Arms support the back with elbows on the floor. Pose should be held a few seconds while breathing freely.

In the Plow pose, legs are lowered over the head until toes touch the floor. Keep knees straight. Hold a few seconds. To lower legs forward until they reach the floor, press down on palms for support. Repeat twice.

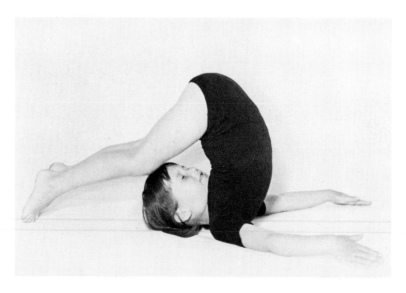

90. THE BOW

In this symbolic pose, the body becomes a bow and the arms are taut bowstrings. The Bow is a good exercise for children and adults. It tones the limbs, slenderizes the waistline, and makes the spine more supple.

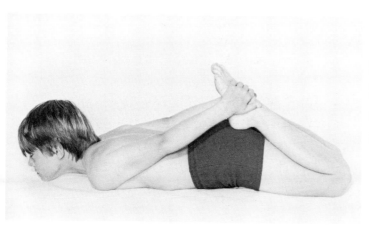

Lie face down, chin touching floor, legs outstretched and together, arms to sides. Bend knees and hold on to ankles.

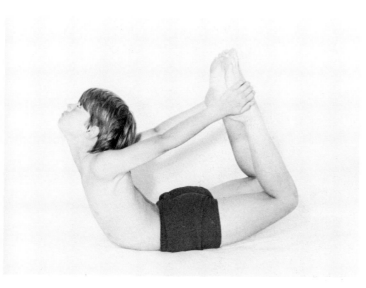

Inhale; raise head, chest and knees off the floor as arms pull tautly. Breathe freely and hold pose a few seconds to feel pull in the spine. Head looks up with throat stretched. Then lower body. Repeat twice.

When this exercise is done with control, rock back and forth about five times as arms pull tautly on legs.

91. THE ARC

This ballet-like pose increases elasticity of the spine, limbers and tones the legs, and develops better balance and muscular control. Children with flexible spines can easily bend backward. Their problem is generally one of balance.

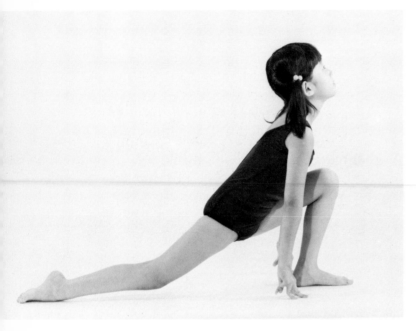

Kneel on left knee. Stretch right leg back as far as possible. Inhale; raise hands overhead and slowly bend backward. Exhale.

Place palms together with head back. Breathe freely and hold pose a few seconds.

Repeat, stretching left leg back.

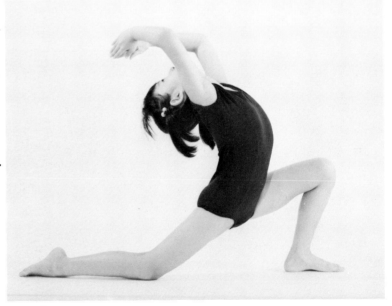

92. THE DIVING SWAN

Children with supple spines are able to achieve this graceful pose in a matter of weeks — some even immediately. The deep backward curve of the spine with toes touching the head gives the body a complete stretch. *Do not force the body into this pose.*

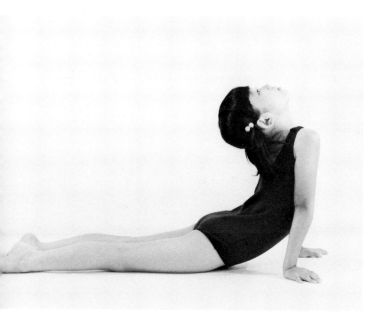

Lie face down with legs together, arms bent with palms flat on floor. Inhale; raise torso to arch the spine with arms fully outstretched.

Breathe freely. Bend legs up toward head. Bend head back until head and toes touch.

Repeat three times.

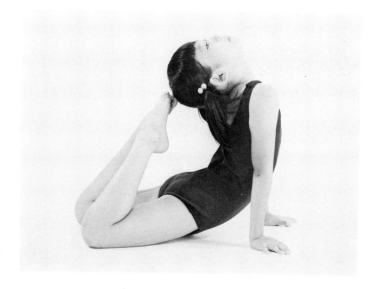

93. THE ARCHER

Also called The Shooting Bow, this stretching posture is less complicated than it appears. Limber children have no difficulty with it. They like to imagine that they are little archers in action. For the less limber child, this exercise should be taught in gradual stages. First practice Step 1 to give the muscles time to stretch; then combine it with Step 2. The breathing is free.

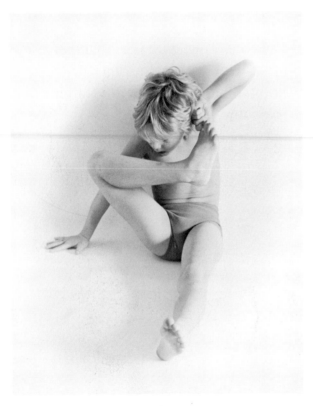 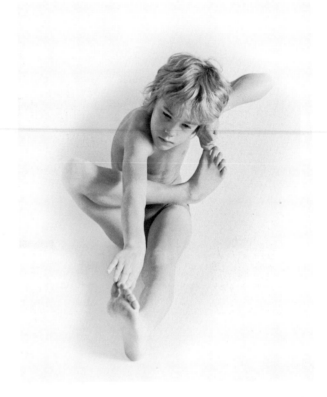

Sit with legs outstretched. Bend right leg and bring it up near the left ear. Grasp the big toe with the left hand.

Bend forward and grasp the big toe of the left foot with the right hand, or hold on to the foot. The right arm crosses over the right leg. Hold the pose a few seconds to feel the stretch. Relax. Repeat, bringing left leg up near right ear.

94. THE TREE

This is an exercise for balance, posture and concentration. Some children are able to do it immediately, while others may need some practice.

The Tree should be practiced near a support for the child whose balance is unsteady. To help maintain his balance, he should concentrate on a fixed object at eye level. This posture is a simplified version of Exercise 30. The breathing is free.

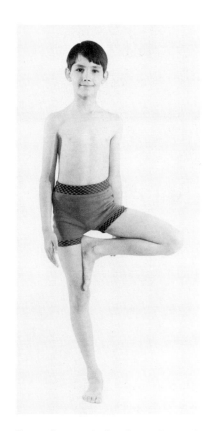 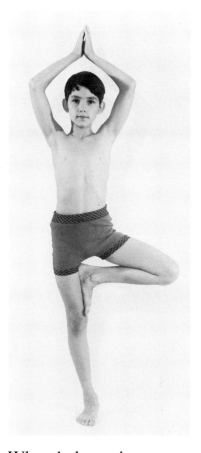 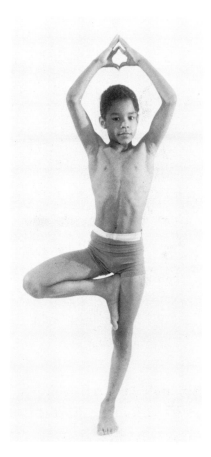

Stand on right leg. Bend left leg so that foot will rest against inner thigh of right leg.

When balance is secure, raise hands overhead with palms or fingertips touching. Hold a few seconds. Relax and

repeat same movements bending right leg so that foot will rest against inner thigh of left leg.

95. THE MOUNTAIN

Though an impressive-looking posture, children with limber legs can do it immediately. Those who are unable to sit in the Lotus pose (described for adults in Exercise 37) should practice the limbering exercise for knees and ankles given in Exercises 5 and 78 (The Sitting Frog).

Sitting in the Lotus pose will keep knees and ankles flexible. The breathing is free.

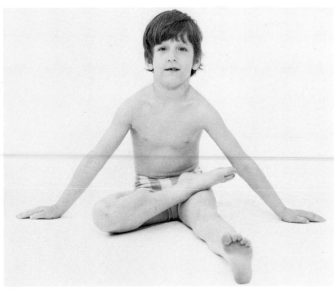

Sit with legs far apart, spine straight, hands to sides with palms down. Bend right leg and bring foot over the left thigh.

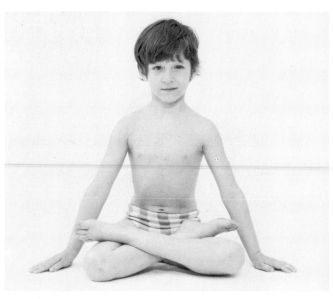

Then bend left leg over the right and bring the foot close to the thigh.

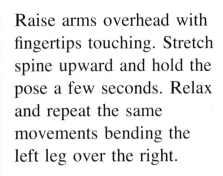

Raise arms overhead with fingertips touching. Stretch spine upward and hold the pose a few seconds. Relax and repeat the same movements bending the left leg over the right.

96. THE LOTUS FISH

Once the Lotus pose is mastered, (Exercise 95, Steps 1 and 2), this posture will be easy to do.

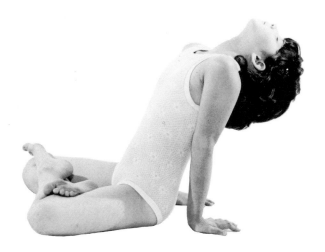

Sit in the Lotus pose: right foot over left thigh, left foot over right thigh. Palms are flat on floor behind back for support.

Inhale; lower back until head touches the floor.

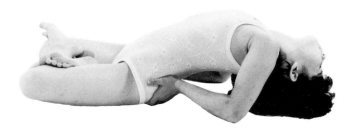

Exhale; arch spine to create a bridge between the head and buttocks. Place palms together over the chest. Breathe freely and hold the pose a few seconds. Relax and repeat the same movements crossing the left leg over the right and right over the left.

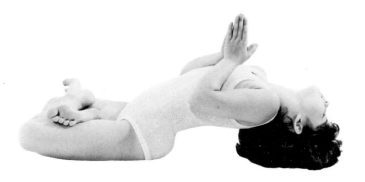

97. THE TORTOISE

This is one of the more difficult yoga postures; it requires a completely limber spine, legs and arms. The forward stretches in Exercise 40 will help in the limbering process for the tight-muscled child.

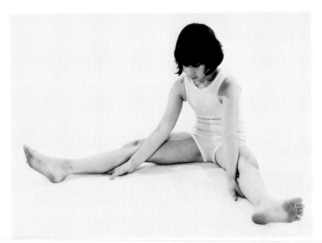 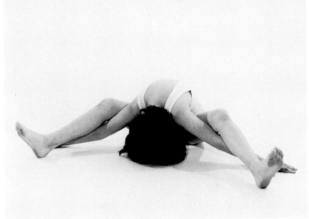

Sit with legs far apart. Inhale; bend forward and extend arms under legs, palms flat on floor.

Exhale; lower head toward floor, *but do not force.* When body becomes

more limber, the head will rest easily on the floor and arms will extend farther back under the legs. Breathe freely and hold the pose a few seconds. Repeat three times, gradually increasing the stretch.

98. THE THUNDERBOLT

This is an exercise of balance and muscle control. Boys take to it naturally. Adults will find it an excellent way to strengthen back muscles and tone buttocks and hips.

Sit with legs together, palms flat on either side of hips. Inhale; press palms down and raise legs up as high as possible, at the same time tilting body backward for balance. Exhale; breathe freely and hold the pose a few seconds. Then lower legs. Repeat three times.

99. THE FISHHOOK

Also known as the Triangle Pose, these side stretches will limber the spine and tone arms, legs and waistline.

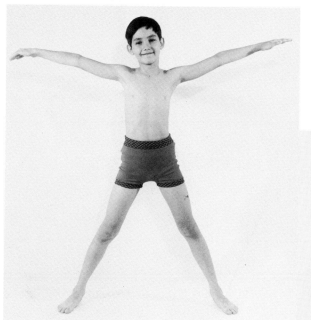

Stand with feet apart and arms outstretched at sides.

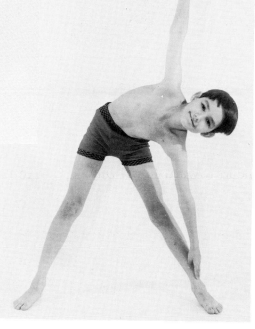

Inhale; bend body to the left side with left arm holding on to the ankle. Right arm is stretched up in line with the left arm.

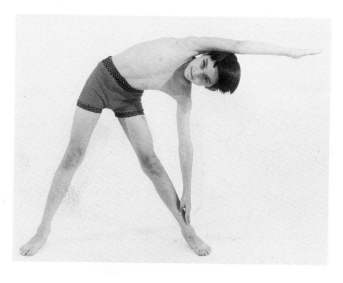

Exhale; extend right arm straight over head to the left. Breathe freely and hold the pose a few seconds to feel stretch along the underside of arm and waist. Relax, then repeat same movements bending to the right side.

100. THE SWIMMER

Children enjoy this exercise, which is similar to the movements of a swimmer with all muscles at work. Adults will find it has a firming effect on the entire body, particularly the abdomen.

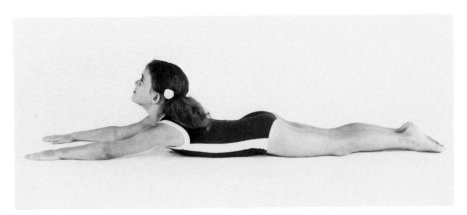

Lie flat, face down, with legs and arms extended, head up.

101. HEADSTAND

Children should be taught the Headstand with caution. The parent who has learned to do it can understand the difficulties one confronts when first practicing this exercise. First of all, the child's head must rest on a thick folded blanket or towel so that there will be no strain on the head. Let him practice "walking in" to the headstand as shown in Steps 3 and 4. When these steps have been mastered, proceed with the next stage. The child will need a little support to get his legs off the floor. Help him by holding his upper thighs. This will enable him to come up gradually into the headstand position. If he is close to a wall, let go for a few seconds

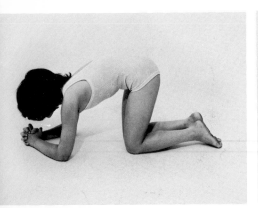
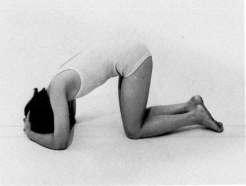
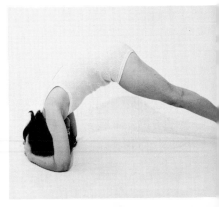

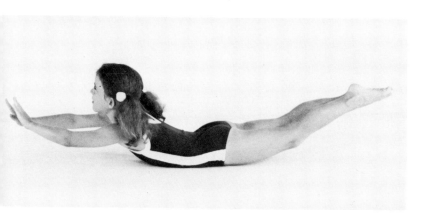

Inhale, at the same time raising arms and legs. Breathe freely, hold a few seconds, then relax. Inhale again, raising arms and legs. While breathing freely, rock back and forth about five times, then relax. Repeat twice.

(but stand close) so that he can test his balance and control. At first his feet will waver back and forth near the wall. Balance will come with continued practice. When coming down from the headstand, reverse the sequence of steps.

If children are taught to *let go* as they fall, their muscles will relax, and in this way they will not injure themselves. See Exercise 43 for detailed explanation of the Headstand.

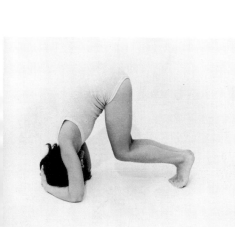

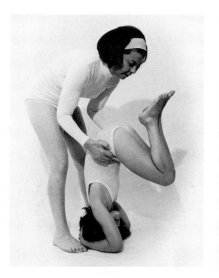

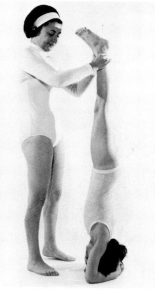

102. TRIPOD HEADSTAND

Many children learn the Tripod Headstand in gym classes. They find it much easier to do than the traditional Headstand.

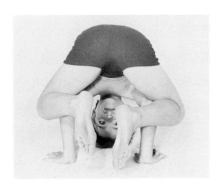

Squat with legs apart, elbows bent and pressing against inner part of knees, palms flat on floor. Lower head to floor.

Slowly raise legs to headstand pose (this should be done close to a wall). When balance is secure—which will take practice—then split legs apart. To come down, join legs, bend knees and lower legs to the floor.

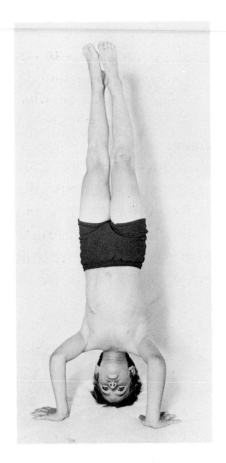

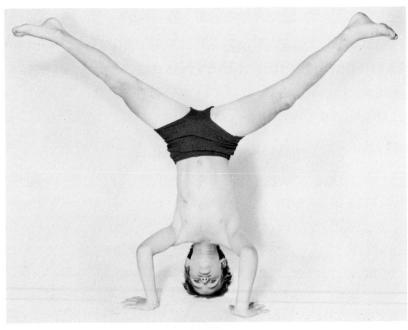

Chapter

6

SIMPLE STEPS TO RELAXING

Have you ever watched a cat relax? Unlike man, animals have the instinctive ability to let go completely. Before a cat settles down to a snooze, it indulges in a long stretch of the body with paws tautly spread out and the back arched, followed by a cavernous yawn which extends even to the tip of the curled tongue. Before it becomes limp and is restfully at ease, it has stretched every muscle in its body.

Man's ability to switch off activity and relax from the cares of the day is a different matter. Many busy people have had to develop their own methods of relaxing in order to replenish their inner reserves. Winston Churchill was known to work long, exhausting hours, yet by retiring for short periods he was able to emerge refreshed; his energy thus replenished, he could become more deliberate in his thoughts and actions.

But many of us, even without Churchill's critical responsibilities, live in a state of constant stress, our energies depleted, our tempers on edge, too keyed up to relax. In desperation, some of us turn to tranquilizing drugs to ease the tension. Yet in each of us nature has provided a built-in tranquilizer which can be activated by deep breathing and muscle stretching.

In yoga we learn to use the power of autosuggestion to consciously relax our muscles. By following a definite sequence of stretching movements, we are able to relax every part of the body, particularly where the points of tension lie.

The first phase in relaxing is to remove or loosen any tight clothing. Then lie on your back with your arms and legs loosely apart. Close your eyes and stretch out to full length. Breathe in deeply (through the nose) and raise your arms over your head. Hold your breath and stretch from head to toe like a cat, tensing all muscles. Then let go and exhale slowly (again through the nose), while you drop your

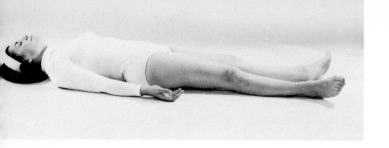

arms limply forward and down. This method of stretching is a good way to wake yourself up in the mornings, and to feel more alert when you wish.

The second step to complete relaxation is to let your imagination take over. As you lie limply at ease, feel as if you are sinking, slowly sinking. Take a long, deep breath and imagine that a flow of energy is saturating your body. Exhale quietly, releasing your breath very slowly.

Then relax your muscles. Starting with your feet, tense them, and let go. Bend your toes down, stretch each one and let go. Now concentrate on each toe and feel it becoming limp. Let your thoughts move gradually to relax the insteps, heels, calves, knees and thighs until your legs feel loose and free. Slowly bend your right knee, sliding your foot along the floor toward you, then let it move back to its relaxed position. Now bend and relax your left knee in the same way. Think of waves of relaxation spreading into your thighs, abdomen, chest, and shoulders; then down into your spine and the small of your back. Feel a tingling sensation as the muscles begin to loosen. Now let your arms and hands become limp. Relax your fingers one by one. Close and open your fists just to feel how relaxed your hands have become.

Next direct your mind to your facial muscles, which we never think of relaxing. Let your jaw sag with lips slightly parted so that your teeth are not clenched. Yawn and stretch the facial muscles. Then feel a loosening of your scalp. Let your eyes sink back into their sockets, resting them in a sea of black silence. The feeling of relaxation is gradually overtaking your whole body. Feel that you are slowly melting away until you are light as air.

Now lie still and become conscious of the steady, slow beating of your heart. Observe your breath as it flows in and out with quiet rhythmic control. Then breathe in deeply and imagine that you are absorbing the forces of energy around you. The inner vibrations of your body are responding to the fresh intake of oxygen. As you breathe out, feel the loosening of tension knots.

Let your mind play steadily on the quiet flow of the breath. Feel that you are dissolving in a state of peace all around you, without clinging to any thoughts. You have now moved into a sphere of serenity, and you are no longer confined within your body. These brief moments of mental refuge will give the mind a rest and induce a mood of tranquillity.

To recharge your energy, take a deep breath and raise your arms up and over your head. Hold your breath and stretch once again like a cat. Repeat the stretch a few times, then slowly come out of the deep relaxation, and you will feel refreshed and revitalized. This is nature's way of recharging your energy and calming your nerves.

The man whose heart and mind are not at rest is without wisdom or the power of contemplation; he who does not practice reflection hath no calm. How can a man without calm obtain happiness?

— The Bhagavad-Gita

Chapter

7

YOGA FOR THE MIND

There is no easy road to instant peace of mind, but our quest for it grows increasingly urgent as the frenetic life-style we pursue allows us no time to pause and reflect. And as our problems become more complex, the pressures more intense, we lose touch with the deeper levels of ourselves. This merry-go-round of activity frequently results in a mental or physical breakdown.

But inner peace cannot be taken by storm. The ways to achieve it are slow.

Through the practice of meditation we can penetrate into the true nature of our being and gain a lasting sense of peace and repose. Since meditation is the direct antithesis of our usual active state, this is an achievement of no small measure.

COMMUNING WITH NATURE

A part of our lives should be spent in the serenity of nature. The Orient knows this, but the West has forgotten it.

How many of us can really enjoy a leisurely walk in the woods or by the seashore without making it into a project?

I recall an evening in Tokyo when a Japanese friend invited me to view the autumn moon, an observance widely practiced in that country. The two of us sat silently absorbing the quiet of her garden. It was a mere fragment of ground, yet a few bronze ornaments, mellowed with the patina of age, were so placed amid the greenery that they enlarged the area, creating a feeling of borrowed scenery. From the weather-beaten bench, we could see the full moon rising as it spread a translucent veil across an arc of dwarfed pines which rustled in the soft breeze.

When we parted that evening, my friend thanked me for sharing the moon with her. We had shared more: peace, stillness, quiet contemplation. And yet the bustling city was just outside the fence.

For those of us who live in crowded cities like New York where the pulse beats at a rapid pace, there is an urgent need for a sense of harmony with nature. We must try to find it wherever we can. Entering into this spiritual harmony of nature is a part of the yogic approach to developing inner calm. By taking a lesson from nature we can enlarge the boundaries of our thoughts. The sky is an example. Its expansiveness does not resist the constant changing of cloud patterns. Think of these clouds as your thoughts and yourself as the clear blue sky. Translate this into a more abstract concept. Since the sky does not resist the clouds, we should accept life's inevitable changes by allowing our thoughts to form new patterns with a mind that is flexible and broad in its horizons.

Many of us would like to practice the art of meditation to develop inner calm, but do not know how. Also, when it comes to the actual discipline of meditation we feel that we simply cannot afford this luxury of time. Our lifestyle does not permit it. But if we could set aside 10 minutes a day for quiet reflection, it would help to bring our thoughts and emotions into focus. Meditation is like a clearinghouse. It puts order into a chaotic mind by sorting out the essentials from nonessentials. We become aware of the whole complex process of life without selecting or rejecting anything. We begin to understand the far-reaching qualities of the mind and to assay the strength we can draw from this sanctuary to reach a calmer mental state.

No beginner is spared the agonies of wrestling with the mind to bar all intruding forces from the quiet flow of thought. In one of my early attempts at meditation, I was unable to shut out the sounds of a struggling violinist. He drove me to despair. But I learned a valuable lesson that day. If we can rise above the noise, absorb it, understand its source and become one with it, the noise will no longer exist.

We can apply this concept to any disturbing force. For instance, if we don't fight pain but try to understand it —

not only how it came about as a personal infliction upon us, but the phenomenon of pain itself and its relation to the total human life — then pain will lose its sting. To achieve this state, one must have highly developed powers of concentration. And before we are able to meditate, we must first learn to concentrate. This is the path of Raja yoga. Its aim is to train the mind so that it will become steady and intensely alive, ready to direct our energies where they are needed.

HOW TO CONCENTRATE

Intense concentration, with the mind turned inward, requires stretches of silence and discipline. In the beginning we will be restless, and seemingly urgent needs will interfere just at the time of concentration. By coaxing the mind gently and diligently, we can direct it back to the point of concentration. Eventually, when we are able to prevent our thoughts from flitting in all directions, it will function with efficiency and calm.

The first step is to select an object for the purpose of concentration. It can be any object — a painting, a sculpture, or a flower. Place the object within close viewing distance. Sit still, and as much as possible try not to fidget. This is a discipline to inculcate mental calm; therefore, the posture chosen must be relaxed and comfortable, with no physical stress on the body. There is no need to sit in a cross-legged yoga posture unless you are used to it. Sitting in a chair with your feet touching the floor and your hands completely relaxed, your back straight but not rigid, is the ideal posture for most of us. The different meditative sitting postures are described in Chapter 2, pages 66–67.

Now you are ready to develop your powers of concentration — but be sure that you are completely relaxed.

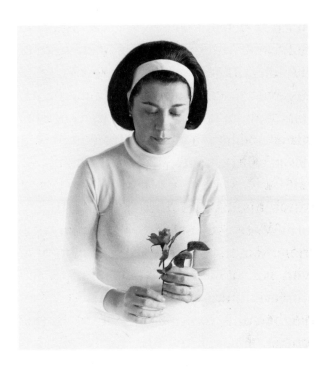

If the object is a flower — say, a fresh red rose — hold it close enough so you can train your entire attention on it. Saturate your senses with its fragrance, texture, form, and color. Gaze at the flower steadily and notice how the petals are held together by the calyx and cupped to embrace one another. Observe the subtle, almost imperceptible shadings of its soft color; the strength of its stem; the richness of its leaves. This may take a minute of intense concentration. Then close your eyes and in your mind's eye recall every feature of the rose. Each time your mind strays, coax it back gently and refocus it on the image of the rose until it is imprinted as vividly as though you were actually looking at it.

The yogis prefer to use a lighted candle as the object of concentration, because they believe the flame stimulates nerve centers in the brain and brings concentration more rapidly.

To practice this gazing exercise, place the candle at eye level and gaze at the flame as long as you can without blinking. Then close your eyes, relax the eye muscles, and envision the flame. Think about its luminous light, its orange glow, and how it emerges from the wick. Think of the candle itself—its shape, its color, and its texture. Concentrate steadily until the image is firmly imprinted in your mind.

Through these exercises you will find your powers of concentration and observation greatly heightened. When you are able to think only of the chosen object and narrow the focus of your mental vision to observe and remember it in the smallest detail, then you will have achieved the height of concentration and will be ready to move into meditation.

HOW TO MEDITATE

If we can think of meditation as a pleasurable experience, we will find moments of great calm even during brief interludes of mental retreat. Through meditation we can resurrect the whole system of our inner life, giving us a fresh point of view and a new source of energy of which we are not ordinarily conscious.

It is possible to meditate at any time and any place, but we should not rush through these precious minutes and expect immediate results. Many of us find that when we sit down to meditate there is a chaos of irrelevant thoughts which come upon us with tremendous force, shattering whatever calm we may feel. The steps to still this inner clamor and bring about a continuous flow of thought take discipline and daily practice. First of all, the mind must be free of any bodily stress. It is important to sit comfortably in a chair or, if you are used to it, on the floor in one of the meditative yoga postures.

Begin by taking long, deep breaths. As you breathe in and out through your nostrils with your eyes closed, be conscious of the movements and changes of your breathing rhythm. Breathe with your whole body. When the cool air reaches your nostrils, feel it entering deep into your lungs and expanding your chest. When the warm air leaves your body, deflating your lungs, feel the process of exhalation. To focus your mind more intently on your breathing rhythm, count each breath slowly up to 20 or 30. While breathing, think of the rhythm as a slow, uninterrupted musical cadence that, as it rises and falls, maintains a steadiness of mood. The moment you are able to lose yourself in the rhythm of your breathing, you will forget your surroundings and tension will slowly melt away.

You can apply all the different

breathing patterns described in Chapter 2 to help calm the mind.

Since the human temperament varies, some of us will respond more quickly than others to the different techniques used in mind control. We should never make any violent attempt to harness the mind—even if it feels like an ocean of storms. If you simply watch your mind without restricting it, the rambling energies of thoughts chasing one another in wild fury will cease. Observe the parade of thoughts that come and go. The pattern will seem like a frisky monkey jumping back and forth. Try to feel the stillness within you and the restlessness of your mind will subside by itself.

Meditate on the concept that your mind is a lake and that your actions are vibrations quivering over the surface. If the surface is smooth, without even a ripple, then you can see the image of your true self reflected on its unbroken surface.

You can also meditate on the five essential principles in yogic philosophy which lead to a higher mental plane. These, in order, are *silence*, to still the mind so that thoughts can enter; *listening*, so that we can learn; *remembering*, so that we can become more considerate; *understanding*, so that our actions will have more meaning; and then *acting*, through performance of everyday duties with a gentle heart and understanding mind.

When our heart becomes more expansive, our outlook free of bias, and we are able to forgive those who have harmed us, then we can truly say that we have progressed on the mental path of yoga.

This leads to creative thinking, which develops inward growth and an awareness of ourselves. We can live a rich, full life if we know how to channel our abilities and talents with the mind silently holding the reins. We should make it a daily habit to turn inward to ourselves and meditate on our inner resources. This is the time to assess our good points, draw from them, develop them. And by becoming aware of the reasons for our failures we will be able to correct them, or at least understand them. By believing in ourselves we expand the limits of our abilities, and by thinking positively we engender strength from within and attract it from without.

There is an enormous chasm between intellectual and spiritual belief. We all feed the need for some guidance to give more meaning to life, particularly when a crisis prevails or when tragedy strikes. In the United Nations building in New York there is a room of quiet where only thoughts speak. In the middle of this dark room, only a shaft of light strikes the surface of a solid rock. This is the symbolic altar dedicated to the God whom man worships under many names and in many forms. There are no other symbols—nothing to distract attention or to break in on the stillness within each person who comes to meditate.

Through the spiritual path of meditation we can all find inner strength. This kind of meditation is like prayer. It floods the soul with sunlight. Every cell of the body, every reflex of the brain is stimulated, filling us with an inner radiance.

To help you meditate spiritually, visualize a burning flame within your heart. That burning flame is the light of the Divine Spirit—the Soul of your soul. When meditating on this light, you will begin to feel a warm glow of serenity. Reading passages from the Bible or repeating a prayer and meditating on the depth of its meaning are other ways to stimulate spiritual awakening.

In a final summary, through patient practice of meditation we learn to discard the weight of fear and worry that bogs us down. We learn to live in the present, without carrying along with us the burdens of the past and unnecessary anxiety over the future. We learn to develop an attitude of nonattachment. Being nonattached does not mean flight from life; rather, it means the ability to view our flaws and potentialities, and to probe the reasons for our failures and successes. We will find peace of mind to give us the strength and vision to accept tragedy and happiness, failure and success with equanimity. As the ancient Chinese proverb says: "If you cannot find it in yourself, where will you go for it?"

Chapter

8

MY FIRST EXPERIENCES WITH YOGA

Looking back twelve years, I remember well that autumn day when I first visited a yoga center in Manhattan. The air was cool and fresh, but I was unable to enjoy it. I suffered from crippling bouts of arthritis and had no hope of cure. Would this, I wondered, be a better formula to limber my joints and soothe my nerves than the standard aid of drugs, hot baths, and a stiff drink to lift my spirits?

The yoga center—this one is no longer in existence, but there are others

—was in an old brownstone. With effort I climbed the steep flight of stairs that led to a reception room where the Swami (spiritual master) greeted me.

"I'm so pleased that you've decided to try yoga," he said. His Indian accent gave his voice a musical cadence.

"Most people do not realize the benefits that yoga brings to the mind and body. Unfortunately, the common belief is that yoga is a highly mystical religion, and in order to practice it one must retreat from life.

"Essentially, in yoga you learn the art of living to keep young and vital. It's as simple as that. I'm sixty-seven, and I've never known what it is—as one says here—to feel old age creeping on."

The Swami was an embodiment of youth and vigor, with an unusually lithe build for a man in his late sixties. His thick dark hair, streaked with gray, fell carelessly about his peaceful face, yet his expression sparkled with vitality. At times he looked boyish.

"How long is the course?" I asked.

"There is no prescribed time. Come as long as you feel the need. But it's important that you practice every day for at least twenty minutes, longer if you can."

I noticed a small wooden box on the wall with boldly written letters that spelled DONATION . . . $1.00. The Swami told me that his center was non-profit, and existed mainly through support from members. I promptly slipped a dollar bill into the slot and walked across the narrow hall to the dressing room. It was small and crowded. A group of women engaged in lively conversation were slipping into tights and leotards. As I looked for an empty space in which to change, a tall, pretty honey-colored blonde cleared a corner for me.

"You're new here, aren't you?" she asked. "What are you in for?"

From the way she phrased her question, I felt I was serving time.

"I have arthritis in my spine and joints," I answered, trying to toss it off lightly.

"You poor thing!"

A spritely silver-haired woman spoke up.

"Well, I'm sure you've come to the right place. I'm Mary," she said, extending a fragile hand. "I've been coming here on and off for years. I used to be a dancer. Believe me, the only way to keep in shape is through yoga.

"How old do you think I am?" she challenged.

"I'd say about fifty-five."

"Guess again."

"Sixty?"

"No, I'm seventy-one," she admitted proudly.

"Come on, Mary," one of the women urged, "show what you can do."

In a flash, Mary was standing on her head. The undulating movements of her firm body showed grace and physical control. We applauded with admiration.

In the *ashram** where the yoga sessions were held, the men and women in the class varied in background, age, race, and religion. Yoga transcends all barriers. Anyone can practice it, and the degree of seriousness is an individual choice.

Mats, one for each class member, were spaced in a line on the floor, and I took my place beside an elderly man of wiry build—a professor of economics. On my right was an attractive model in her thirties who told me that through the practice of meditation and deep breathing she had gained an inner poise and calm

---

* A place where people meet for religious instruction or exercises.

that had been invaluable in her work before the camera.

"After a hard day's work," she said, "I usually do the Shoulderstand and remain in it until I feel the blood coming to the surface of my face. It's really the best beauty treatment anyone can have."

The professor had a beguiling sense of humor and a flair for the dramatic. He remarked somewhat jestingly that the only way he could keep up with his young wife was through the practice of yoga.

"It sure has improved my sex life!" he chuckled, peering at me through horn-rimmed glasses.

An air of tranquillity reigned over the sparsely decorated room. Fresh flowers graced a long polished table near a bronze urn which emitted a delicate fragrance of burning incense, and directly above it hung a colorful painting of Indian sages in meditation. This serene atmosphere was exemplified by the Swami, who entered and seated himself in the Lotus pose in quiet contemplation.

There were twenty in the class. Our sessions began with the practice of silence. The Swami chanted, repeating the Sanskrit word *OM* − OM − OM* in long-drawn-out syllables to produce deep concentration that would help us withdraw our minds from their external environment and turn them inward. This

most sacred word of power is synonymous with the name of the Divine Spirit, or God. By repeating *OM* during meditation, first aloud and then silently, one's powers of concentration are stimulated. We were never given an overdose of mental discipline.

From the Swami's discussions in the weeks that followed, we learned that before we could take up the spiritual practice of yoga we must free our minds of jealousy, anger and hate and dismiss all nonessential clutter. When the mind is clouded with worry and anxiety, the inner brightness of the soul is hidden.

Following meditation, we learned to tap the vital energy of life through deep controlled breathing. At first I found the sudden intake of oxygen a little startling. I experienced a surge of vitality as if I had opened the window for a breath of fresh air; yet the quieting effect it had on my mind was hypnotic. It took some practice before I was able to breathe from the diaphragm without conscious effort—which, surprisingly, is the natural way for very young children to breathe, and also for us when we are asleep.

With practice I was able to ventilate my lungs, which years of smoking had left congested. I eventually lost the desire to smoke. Another victory was over insomnia. When I was able to apply a pattern of deep rhythmic breathing to calm my nerves, I could fall into a restful sleep.

The main part of the yoga sessions was devoted to the physical postures, many of which resemble animals, birds

---

* *OM*, represented also as *AUM*, signifies *A*: Evolution; *U*: Preservation; *M*: Dissolution. Life begins and ends with *OM*.

and insects. By imitating these postures, we learned how to stretch and relax our bodies, and move with grace.

Among my favorites were The Fish and The Swan. They were wonderfully stimulating yet relaxing for my weak spine.

At the close of each session, the Swami's melodious voice suggested we let go completely, to feel deep limpness. The atmosphere was conducive to tranquillity—the shutters partially closed to diffuse the light, and the air cool but not drafty. As I lay on the yoga mat submerged in deep repose, my mind drifted into a climate of serenity. I could hear the Swami quoting from the *Upanishads* of the ancient Indian scriptures, as his voice slowly faded: "May quietness descend upon your limbs, your speech, your breath, your eyes, your ears. May all your senses become clear and strong."

After six months of twice-weekly sessions and daily practice, I felt like a new person. But at first I was impatient with my physical limitations. My knee joints and spine were stubbornly rigid, and disregarding the Swami's advice— *never force the body*—I did, and ended up with muscle strain. For days I limped about until the muscles repaired themselves. From then on I practiced the postures with ease and more mind control, stretching only as far as my muscles would permit. I became aware that yoga cannot be done in a hurry or with an agitated mind.

As my muscle tone improved, so did my posture. My step took on bounce, and a wonderful sensation of well-being stayed with me. The pain in my joints and back, which had plagued me for years, subsided. With relief I discarded the traction device I had used nightly to stretch my spine. I began to respond to the lyrical movements of the postures, and the greatest reward came when one day I could do the Headstand, bend backward with ease, and sit in the Lotus pose. My body felt buoyant and free.

After having achieved the physical discipline of Hatha yoga, I was prepared to move on to the higher realm of Raja yoga, which is concerned with one's inner being. Daily meditation has given me a measure of calm, elevating my spirit and expanding my vision. I have found that yoga must be practiced with determination and with a heart that refuses to become discouraged.

SPECIAL EXERCISE PLANS

THIS SECTION will help vary your daily practice routine. At a quick glance you will be able to follow a series of tone-up exercises designed for various time periods, starting with ten minutes. There are also spot exercises for relieving fatigue, tension, or poor circulation, and others focused on specific problems of various parts of the body.

These charts can also be used as guidelines for working out your own exercise plans. You will find it extremely helpful when coordinating the exercises to do them in the order of standing, sitting and lying positions. It is important to include an all-around tone-up plan and not concentrate exclusively on exercises for specific problem areas. If you sketch or trace the different postures from the book, they can then be pasted on cardboard and used as reference while exercising.

Now it is up to you to organize your program. Early morning is usually the best time for most people, and it will help you start the day feeling fit. If this is inconvenient, find your own time at the same hour each day—when you are not rushed.

Exercising in spurts will do you absolutely no good. Your body requires a daily routine of physical exercises from head to toe to become limber and well-toned. If you are not accustomed to exercising regularly, begin by making minimal demands on your body. Start out with just ten minutes a day until the habit of exercising daily is firmly established. Then gradually build up the time to thirty minutes. This may take a month or longer depending on the individual.

When you wake up, do the Complete Breathing exercise in bed. Feel its full impact of body stretch. Continue with the series of Eye Movements while you are debating with yourself whether or not you should exercise that particular morning. Then sit up and do the Head Roll. Now part of the battle is won. You have already begun your morning exercise. The rest requires some self-control and discipline, but with each day it becomes a little easier. The effort will pay off, and you will begin to feel lithe, vibrant and in tune with yourself.

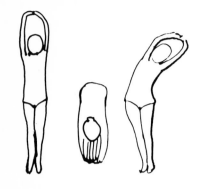

FOUR-WAY STRETCH (P. 33)

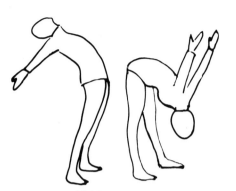

FLIGHT (P. 28)

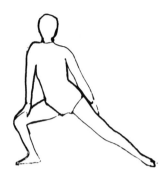

HIP STRETCH (P. 27)

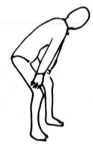

ABDOMINAL LIFT (P. 32)

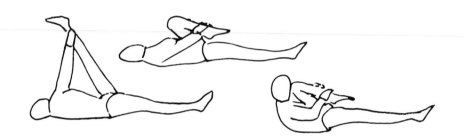

DANCE OF THE LEGS (P. 46)

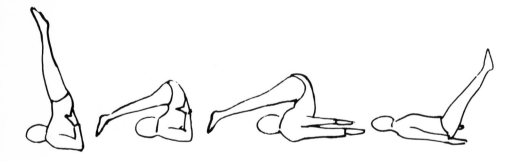

THE SHOULDERSTAND (P. 48)   THE PLOW (P. 77)   THE FISH (P. 119)

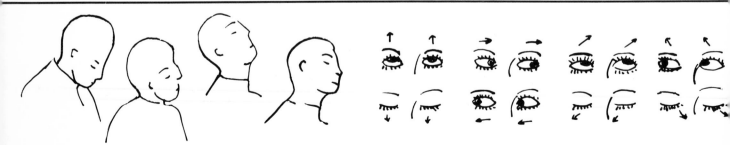

HEAD ROLL (P. 98)   EYE EXERCISES (P. 44)

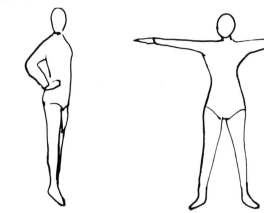

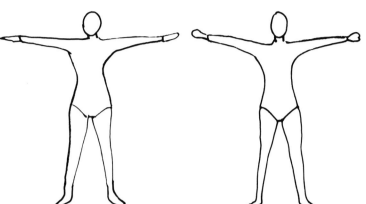

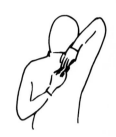

STRENGTHENING FEET
AND ANKLES (P. 26)

FIRMING UNDERSIDES OF ARMS
AND IMPROVING POSTURE (P. 36)

BACK STRETCH (P. 101)

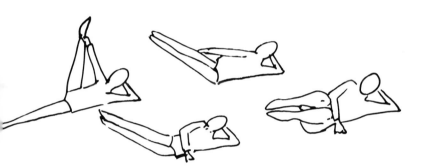

SIDE STRETCHES (P. 56)

ROCKING THE SPINE (P. 25)

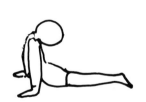

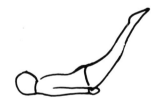

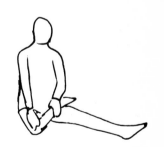

THE COBRA (P. 122)

THE LOCUST (P. 59)

THE BOW (P. 129)

LIMBERING KNEES
AND ANKLES (P. 26)

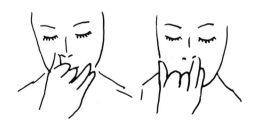

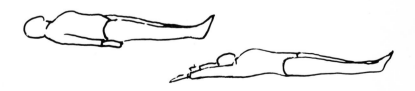

ALTERNATE BREATHING (PP. 42, 54)

COMPLETE BREATHING (P. 23)

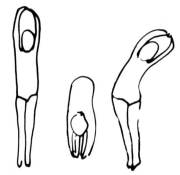
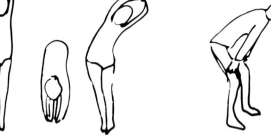
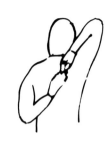

BELLOWS (OR RUNNER'S) BREATH is a dynamic exercise when done while running in place 50 to 100 times. (P. 76)

FOUR-WAY STRETCH (P. 33)   ABDOMINAL LIFT (P. 32)   BACK STRETCH (P. 101)

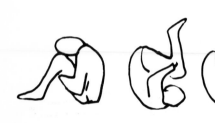
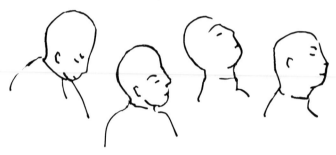

ROCKING THE SPINE (P. 25)   HEAD ROLL (P. 98)

30-MINUTE TONE-UP PLAN

Combine 10-Minute Tone-Up Plan with chart at right.
Substitute more difficult exercises for ones you can already do.

MONDAY

1. Sun Salutation (p. 71)
2. Body Roll (p. 24)
3. The Stoop (p. 55)
4. Side Stretches (p. 56)
5. Inclined Plane (p. 58)
6. The Locust (p. 59)
7. The Wheel (p. 80)
8. The Arc (p. 130)
9. Shoulderstand and Plow Variations (pp. 48, 60, 77)
10. Headstand or First Steps to Headstand (pp. 50, 82)
11. Eye Exercises (while relaxing on back) (p. 44)

TUESDAY

Sun Salutation (p. 71)
Head-to-Knee Stretch (p. 41)
The Tree (p. 63)
Spinal Twist (p. 62)
Forward Bend (p. 69)
Dancer's Pose (p. 92)
The Cobra (p. 122)
The Crow (p. 96)
Shoulderstand and Plow Variations (pp. 48, 60, 77)
Headstand or First Steps to Headstand (pp. 50, 82)
Eye Exercises (p. 44)

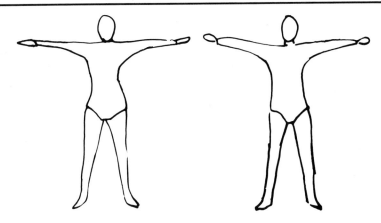

FIRMING UNDERSIDES OF ARMS
AND IMPROVING POSTURE (P. 36)

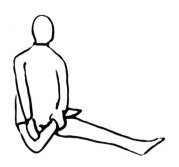

LIMBERING KNEES
AND ANKLES (P. 26)

ALTERNATE BREATHING (PP. 42, 54)

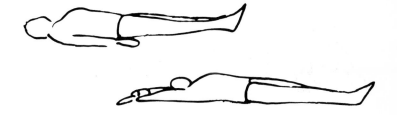

COMPLETE BREATHING (P. 23)

WEDNESDAY	THURSDAY	FRIDAY
Sun Salutation (p. 71)	Sun Salutation (p. 71)	Sun Salutation (p. 71)
Flight (p. 28)	Hip Stretch (p. 27)	Flight (p. 28)
The Arrow (p. 79)	One Leg Stand (p. 95)	Vertical Stretch and Knee Bend (p. 37)
Deep Knee Bend (p. 94)	Thunderbolt (p. 136)	The Eagle (p. 94)
Dance of the Legs (p. 46)	The Swan (p. 124)	Spinal Balance (p. 62)
Side Stretches (p. 56)	The Bridge (p. 46)	The Fish (pp. 93, 119)
The Bow (p. 129)	Leg Splits (p. 78)	The Camel (p. 34)
The Archer (p. 132)	The Tortoise (p. 136)	The Swimmer (p. 138)
Shoulderstand and Plow Variations (pp. 48, 60, 77)	Shoulderstand and Plow Variations (pp. 48, 60, 77)	Shoulderstand and Plow Variations (pp. 48, 60, 77)
Headstand or First Steps to Headstand (pp. 50, 82)	Headstand or First Steps to Headstand (pp. 50, 82)	Headstand or First Steps to Headstand (pp. 50, 82)
Eye Exercises (p. 44)	Eye Exercises (p. 44)	Eye Exercises (p. 44)

Note: Use any two columns for Saturday and Sunday.

EXERCISES TO ELIMINATE FATIGUE AND TENSION

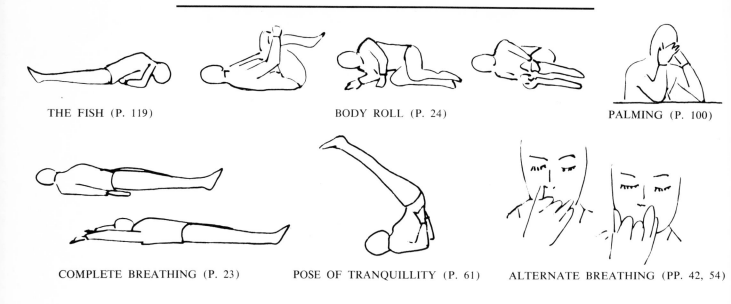

THE FISH (P. 119)　　　　BODY ROLL (P. 24)　　　　PALMING (P. 100)

COMPLETE BREATHING (P. 23)　　　POSE OF TRANQUILLITY (P. 61)　　　ALTERNATE BREATHING (PP. 42, 54)

EXERCISES TO STIMULATE CIRCULATION AND INTESTINAL ACTIVITY

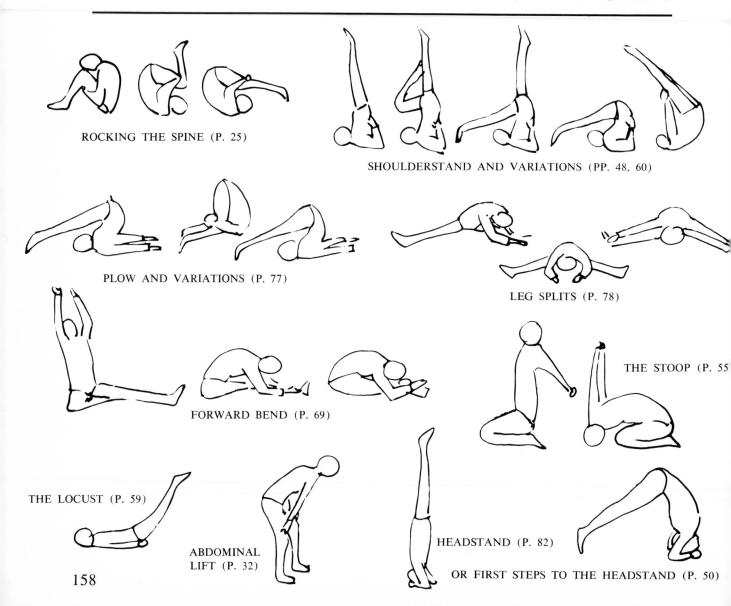

ROCKING THE SPINE (P. 25)

SHOULDERSTAND AND VARIATIONS (PP. 48, 60)

PLOW AND VARIATIONS (P. 77)

LEG SPLITS (P. 78)

FORWARD BEND (P. 69)

THE STOOP (P. 55

THE LOCUST (P. 59)

ABDOMINAL LIFT (P. 32)

HEADSTAND (P. 82)

OR FIRST STEPS TO THE HEADSTAND (P. 50)

EXERCISES FOR SPECIFIC NEEDS

INDEX